Sara Miller McCune founded SAGE Publishing in 1965 to support the dissemination of usable knowledge and educate a global community. SAGE publishes more than 1000 journals and over 800 new books each year, spanning a wide range of subject areas. Our growing selection of library products includes archives, data, case studies and video. SAGE remains majority owned by our founder and after her lifetime will become owned by a charitable trust that secures the company's continued independence.

Los Angeles | London | New Delhi | Singapore | Washington DC | Melbourne

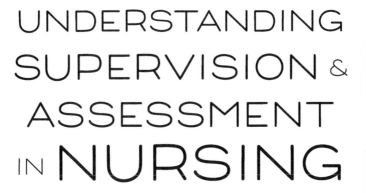

UNDERSTANDING SUPERVISION & ASSESSMENT IN NURSING

ÁINE FEENEY & SUZANNE EVERETT

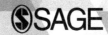

Los Angeles | London | New Delhi
Singapore | Washington DC | Melbourne

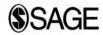

Los Angeles | London | New Delhi
Singapore | Washington DC | Melbourne

SAGE Publications Ltd
1 Oliver's Yard
55 City Road
London EC1Y 1SP

SAGE Publications Inc.
2455 Teller Road
Thousand Oaks, California 91320

SAGE Publications India Pvt Ltd
B 1/I 1 Mohan Cooperative Industrial Area
Mathura Road
New Delhi 110 044

SAGE Publications Asia-Pacific Pte Ltd
3 Church Street
#10-04 Samsung Hub
Singapore 049483

Editor: Alex Clabburn
Assistant editor: Jade Grogan
Production editor: Tanya Szwarnowska
Copyeditor: Jane Robson
Proofreader: Brian McDowell
Indexer: Avril Ehrlich
Marketing manager: George Kimble
Cover design: Wendy Scott
Typeset by: C&M Digitals (P) Ltd, Chennai, India
Printed in the UK

Library of Congress Control Number: 2019943676

British Library Cataloguing in Publication data

A catalogue record for this book is available
from the British Library.

ISBN 978-1-5264-6803-1
ISBN 978-1-5264-6802-4 (pbk)

At SAGE we take sustainability seriously. Most of our products are printed in the UK using responsibly sourced
papers and boards. When we print overseas we ensure sustainable papers are used as measured by the
PREPS grading system. We undertake an annual audit to monitor our sustainability.

CONTENTS

ABOUT THE AUTHORS

Su Everett, RN, BSc (Hons); MSc; PG Cert (HE), is a Senior Lecturer at Middlesex University and Senior Teaching Fellow. She works as a Senior Practitioner at the Royal Free Hospital in sexual health.

Áine Feeney, RN, BSc (Hons); MA in practice education, is a Senior Lecturer at Middlesex University and has an interest in practice education.

AUTHORS'
ACKNOWLEDGEMENTS

We would like to thank Kathy Wilson, Nora Cooper and the staff in the Practice Based Learning Unit at Middlesex University.

PUBLISHER'S ACKNOWLEDGEMENTS

The Publishers would like to thank Peter Ellis, Karen Elcock, Gary Witham and Zoe Broad for the editorial input at various stages of the book's development.

Appendix 1 and 2 have been reproduced in full from the NMC Standards for nurses in line with their terms and conditions. Modifications have been made to text style and layout only. No changes have been made to the text and full versions of these documents can be found at: www.nmc.org.uk/standard

1

INTRODUCTION TO THE 2018 NMC STANDARDS FOR NURSES AND MIDWIVES

AIMS OF THIS CHAPTER

- To understand the different components of the NMC Standards of proficiency for registered nurses
- To develop an initial understanding of the five headings used in the Standards framework for nursing and midwifery education
- To understand the key titles and roles within student practice learning
- To develop an initial understanding of the Standards for student supervision and assessment.

Introduction

In 2018 the Nursing and Midwifery Council produced new standards of proficiency for registered nurses. These were outlined in two sets of standards. The first set are *Future Nurse: Standards of Proficiency for Registered Nurses* which detail the knowledge, skills and attributes students need to demonstrate in order to successfully become registered nurses. The second set of standards provides an education framework called *Realising Professionalism: Standards for Education and Training*. This sets the standards required for education and training (NMC, 2018a) and is to be utilised by Approved Education Institutes (AEIs) in conjunction with practice placement and work placed partners to ensure that the quality of training meets the NMC's standards.

This book has been written for anyone who is new to the 2018 NMC Standards with an involvement in student practice learning. It provides a short introduction that seeks to elaborate on the standards and provide some guidance on how they can be implemented effectively. It focuses on practice learning so will be useful for anyone taking on a supervision role for the first time or those looking to quickly understand the new system of practice learning. The book focuses primarily on practice learning of pre-registration student nurses, although much of the discussion will be equally relevant for other health professions.

There are three parts to *Realising Professionalism: Standards for Education and Training* which must be utilised together. These are:

- Part 1: Standards framework for nursing and midwifery education (NMC, 2018a)
- Part 2: Standards for student supervision and assessment (NMC, 2018b)
- Part 3: Programme standards (NMC, 2018c).

Parts 1 and 2 are most relevant for practice supervisors and assessors and we will now provide a short overview of these to help contextualise the subsequent chapters. Abridged versions of both these documents are available in the appendix section at the back of the book.

Part 1: Standards framework for nursing and midwifery education

The NMC has broken the standards framework down into five headings (see Figure 1.1) which outline the requirements of all teaching programmes approved by the NMC. These headings apply to the theoretical learning and learning in the practice placement and workplaced areas.

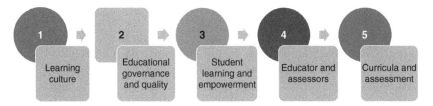

Figure 1.1 The five headings of the Standards framework for nursing and midwifery education

The following activity will help you reflect on the headings used by the NMC.

ACTIVITY 1.1

Reflection on the Standards framework for nursing and midwifery education

Write short notes on each heading setting out what you think each one means.

In the NMC's Standards framework each heading addresses an aspect of education (NMC, 2018a). This book has taken each heading separately and focused a chapter on it, discussing the NMC requirements and how these should be addressed in approved educational institutes and practice-based learning. We will now briefly describe each of the five headings in turn.

Heading 1: learning culture

—————— STANDARDS ——————

S1.1   Learning culture prioritises the safety of people including carers, students and educators, and enables the values of *The Code* to be upheld (NMC, 2018a).

S1.2   Education and training is valued in all learning environments (NMC, 2018a).

What do these standards mean?

Heading 1 asks educational institutes and practice placements and work placed learning partners to put the safety of the people we care for at the forefront. It emphasises the importance of students and educators recognising and raising concerns, encouraging an open and honest environment. This emphasises health professionals' duty of candour which involves being transparent about mistakes to service users. It also links to whistleblowing and raising concerns.

This heading says that a learning culture should be diverse and free of discrimination. Feedback should be sought from students, educators and service users and acted upon. Education institutes, practice placements and work placed learning partners should all collaborate to ensure that inter-professional learning is embraced and opportunities to work together to improve education and service provision should be sought through evidence-based research.

Heading 2: educational governance and quality

──────────────── STANDARDS ────────────────

S2.1 Approved education institutions and their practice placement and work placed partners have effective governance systems that ensure compliance with all legal, regulatory, professional and educational requirements, with clear lines of responsibility and accountability for meeting those requirements and responding when standards are not met (NMC, 2018a).

S2.2 Approved education institutions and their practice placement and work placed partners optimise safety and ensure quality, taking account of the diverse needs of, and working in partnership with, students, service users, carers and all other stakeholders (NMC, 2018a).

What do these standards mean?

The NMC states that approved education institutes and practice placement and work based learning partners communicate with each other and share responsibility for the delivery, development and evaluation of programmes. There should be fairness and transparency in the selection and recruitment of students, and impartial fitness to practise procedures for students.

A safe environment should be provided for learning, and this should safely provide learning opportunities and practical experience for students. To ensure quality and safety of programmes these should adhere to standards and requirements set by the NMC, and suitably qualified and experienced people should be programme leaders delivering this learning.

Heading 3: student learning and empowerment

———————— STANDARDS ————————

S3.1   Students are provided with a variety of learning opportunities and appropriate resources which enable them to achieve their learning outcomes, NMC proficiencies and be capable of demonstrating the professional behaviours in *The Code* (NMC, 2018a).

S3.2   Students are empowered and supported to become resilient, caring, reflective and lifelong learners who are capable of working in inter-professional and multi-agency teams (NMC, 2018a).

What do these standards mean?

Students should be supported through theory and practice, with inductions, timely information on practice placements and curriculum, and assessments all provided. Students should be allocated and have access to a nominated practice assessor and nominated academic assessor for each programme.

Students should be empowered by approved education institutes, practice placement and work placed learning partners. They should be encouraged to be responsible for their well-being and protected from behaviour which undermines their physical and mental health.

Heading 4: educators and assessors

—————————————— **STANDARDS** ——————————————

S4.1   Theory and practice learning and assessment are facilitated effectively and impartially by appropriately qualified and experienced professionals with necessary expertise for their educational roles (NMC, 2018a).

What does this standard mean?

All educators and assessors must act as role models and adhere to the NMC requirements. They should have access to ongoing training and induction. They should have supported time and resources to fulfil their roles. They should have access to feedback from students about their roles.

Heading 5: curricula and assessment

—————————————— **STANDARDS** ——————————————

S5.1   Curricula and assessments are developed, implemented and reviewed to ensure that students achieve the learning outcomes and NMC proficiencies for their approved programme (NMC, 2018a).

What does this standard mean?

The curriculum should adhere to NMC requirements. The curriculum should be structured, developing in complexity. Assessments should be reliable and valid. Assessment in practice is based on indirect and direct observation. Students should receive objective feedback in theory and practice during their programmes.

Part 2: Standards for student supervision and assessment (NMC 2018b)

The Nursing and Midwifery Council has produced a second document on guidance for standards for education and training (NMC, 2018b).

This has created new titles and roles: 'practice assessor' instead of 'mentor', 'practice supervisor' and finally the 'academic assessor' which is similar to 'programme leader'. Nursing students will be assigned to practice and academic assessors who are registered nurses with appropriate equivalent experience for the student's field of practice (NMC, 2018b). Midwifery students will be assigned to practice and academic assessors who are registered midwives (NMC, 2018b).

The role of the practice assessor

The higher education institute and practice learning area must support practice assessors to prepare and support the assessment of students. They should provide constructive feedback to facilitate professional development of students and understand the proficiencies and the programme outcomes that students need to achieve (NMC, 2018b).

The role of the practice supervisors

Practice supervisors contribute to the ongoing observation, training and assessment of students (NMC, 2018b). All registered nurses and midwives can supervise students, acting as role models for safe and effective practice. Students may be supervised by other registered health and social care professionals.

The role of the academic assessors

The role of the academic assessor is to confirm the student's achievement and proficiencies for each part of their nurse training. This will be based on the student's knowledge and expertise and their conduct, with communication between academic and practice assessors. Academic assessors cannot be the practice supervisor and practice assessor for the same student.

The *Standards of Proficiency for Registered Nurses* (NMC, 2018d) outline the role of the nurse in the 21st century, the future nurse. As there had been eight years since the introduction of the previous documents – *Standards for Pre-Registration Nursing Education* (NMC, 2010a) and *Standards for Competence for Registered Nurses* (NMC, 2010b) – nurse education was due an overhaul of how to train, educate, supervise and assess student nurses for graduate entry to the nursing register.

The previous standards (NMC, 2010b) were outlined under four aspects:

- Professional values
- Communication and interpersonal skills
- Nursing practice and decision-making, and
- Leadership, management and team working

In addition to these aspects were competencies for nurses from all fields and other field-specific competencies. Combining both areas and these competencies the NMC was confident that patients and the public could be confident in registered nurses (NMC, 2010b). These documents continue to identify the differences between the fields of nursing and the competence expectations related to each field, including the common competencies listed above.

With the introduction of the new standards (NMC, 2018d) there are significant changes to the competencies and the skills to be achieved by all fields of nursing. All competencies are relevant to all fields, with different levels of knowledge and skill required dependent on field. The proficiencies have now been structured with seven platforms followed by two annexes.

The platforms are:

1. Being an accountable professional
2. Promoting health and preventing ill health
3. Assessing needs and planning care
4. Providing and evaluating care
5. Leading and managing nursing care and working in teams
6. Improving safety and quality of care
7. Coordinating care

The annexes indicate the skills and procedures registered nurses should be able to demonstrate, with more advanced skills identified for registered nurses working in particular fields of practice.

These annexes identify a significant number of skills and procedures required at the point of registration. There have been a number of additional skills included in this version of the standards that aim to assist practice and the registered nurse on qualifying. These include:

- Venepuncture/cannulation and blood sampling
- Chest auscultation
- Rectal examination and manual evacuation.

Another significant change with the standards introduced in 2018 is the introduction of the new supervision, assessor and academic assessor roles to replace the previous role of the mentor (NMC, 2008). Chapter 2 on educators and assessors discussed these roles.

Although it will be the responsibility of approved education institutions to make sure students achieve these competencies and skills, it is important that practice supervisors and assessors have a broad understanding of what students are working towards. You are advised to familiarise yourself with the 'Standards of proficiency for registered nurses' which can found on the NMC website (www.nmc.org.uk/standards/standards-for-nurses/).

CHAPTER SUMMARY

In this chapter we have:

- Introduced the new standards from the NMC
- Discussed the changes and how these will affect students
- Discussed the changes and how these affect practice supervisors and assessors and their roles.

2

UNDERSTANDING THE DIFFERENT ROLES WITHIN PRACTICE EDUCATION

Educators and assessors

S4.1 Theory and practice learning and assessment are facilitated effectively and impartially by appropriately qualified and experienced professionals with the necessary expertise for their educational roles.

AIMS OF THIS CHAPTER

- To understand the role of the educator
- To understand the role of the practice supervisor
- To understand the role of the practice assessor
- To understand the role of the academic assessor
- To embrace the resources available to educators and assessors for supporting learners in practice
- To learn to utilise student feedback to enhance the educators' and assessors' development.

Introduction

Clinical practice education is provided both theoretically and practically. All higher education institutions (HEIs) will have lecture/seminar-based teaching sessions complemented with practice-based skills sessions in customised skills laboratories. Health education is constituted of many theoretical components and these are taught and assessed at an academic level within the respective HEI. Students will attend lectures and seminars and will be regularly assessed through assignments, tests and exams. When it comes to the practical component of their education assessment largely takes place in the clinical area. Pre-registration nurse education continues to be constituted of 50 per cent theoretical learning and 50 per cent practical learning (NMC, 2018a), making collaboration between HEIs and clinical employers/clinical placement providers essential in order to complete the process of assessment. There are various ways to meet the practical element of the programme, including simulated practice carried out at the HEI in support of the practice-based learning carried out in the clinical area.

The role of the educator

For the purpose of this book the term 'educator' will be used to refer to both the academic educator teaching students theory-based learning at the HEI and those who contribute to the learning that takes place within the practice setting. In 2018 the NMC (2018a) introduced changes to the education framework in relation to learning and assessment for all nursing and midwifery programmes. There are now three distinct roles relating to learning and assessment in the practice setting. These are: practice supervisors, practice assessors and an academic assessor. These roles need to be adequately prepared for. Anyone moving into a supervisor role must be a registered health and social care professional – this may include, nurses, doctors, physiotherapists, operating department practitioners, etc. The practice assessor must be a registered nurse or midwife who has been suitably prepared to undertake the role. The practice supervisor and practice assessor cannot be the same individual. This is a very significant distinction designed to make the assessment of students' practical skills more robust. Finally, the academic assessor must also be a registered nurse or midwife from an approved education institution (AEI) working in partnership with the practice placement. Table 2.1 separates out these different roles and the requirements. It is important to note that the practice assessor and the academic assessor need to be nominated individuals. This change in delivery of supervision and assessment is aimed at providing more consistency and objectivity to the assessment process. Duffy (2003) discussed the advantages of separating the roles rather than having an individual mentor responsible for both teaching and assessing students in practice.

Table 2.1   Requirements for learning and assessment support of students in practice.

Who	Professional registration requirements	Education and support
Practice Supervisor	Registered health and social care professional	Understanding of the role – including their observations contributing to the assessment process
Practice Assessor (nominated)	Registered nurse or midwife	Suitably prepared with ongoing support
Academic Assessor (nominated)	Registered nurse or midwife	Suitably prepared with ongoing support

Practice supervisor

The practice supervisor of a student in clinical practice is there to enable the student to learn and safely achieve proficiency and autonomy in their developing professional role (NMC, 2018a). The practice supervisor participates in one of the roles of educator in clinical practice. The practice supervisor does not necessarily need to be a registered nurse – this role is available to other registered health and social care professionals. This includes nursing associates, social workers and other registered professionals from the multi-professional team. This enables student nurses to be supervised in a wide range of practice areas that were previously not widely available due to the limited availability of registered nurse/mentors. If you are not registered with a professional regulator then you cannot be a practice supervisor. However, not being registered does not stop you from contributing to the learning of a student in your clinical environment. There are experiences, skills and other competencies that non-registered professionals can contribute where learning is taking place, e.g. working with teachers, phlebotomists, managers, and the system is intended to allow for dynamic learning opportunities drawing on the rich pool of knowledge held across the healthcare team.

Students will be appropriately supervised during their placement in a way that reflects their learning needs and the stage of their learning. For instance, a first year student on their first clinical placement will need a different level of supervision to a final year student nearing the point of registration. Completion of orientation and initial meetings to review the student's practice documentation will help to establish the needs and expectations that are right for the level of the student. Practice documentation is a key tool for the practice supervisor to be familiar with. This document will outline the student's stage of learning, the competencies still to be achieved, both professional and clinical, and provide the student, their assessor and future supervisors with valuable information on their continuing development.

A practice supervisor needs to be current in their own area of practice and act as a role model for the student under their supervision. There must be adherence to their own code of conduct related to their registration. Providing support, supervision and feedback is an essential element of the practice supervisor role. Students require feedback to support their learning, to understand where they need to improve and enhance the care and service that they are providing (Walsh, 2014).

Preparation of the practice supervisor

Approved education institutions and their practice partners need to jointly support practice supervisors. Preparation of practice supervisors must include ongoing support to prepare, reflect on and develop effective supervision. The practice supervisor will also be a vital contributor to the student's learning and assessment. As part of their initial preparation practice supervisors must also have an understanding of what the student is expected to achieve through proficiencies and programme outcomes.

Supervision of a student/learner in your environment will depend on a number of factors. The level of supervision required of the learner will be determined on an individual basis. Practice supervisors need to have an understanding of the proficiencies a learner requires and these will differ depending on

- The type of learner
- The individual student
- Their stage of learning

- The placement
- The practice supervisor's role in education of students.

Support, training and education need to be in place for supervisors. However, this intervention will depend on the practice supervisor's previous experience. Practice supervisors have a responsibility to identify their own individual learning needs in order to support students. Previous experience of supporting students is beneficial in becoming a practice supervisor; this could include previous formal training or 'on the job' training. The AEIs have a responsibility to ensure that the correct support, education and training are provided so that all preparation of supervisors upholds public protection (NMC, 2018b).

All nominated practice supervisors must meet the NMC (2018c) standards on supervision of students. The AEIs together with practice partners must ensure that practice supervisors receive ongoing support in relation to preparation, reflection on and development of effective supervision and contribute to student learning and assessment. As part of their preparation practice supervisors must have an understanding of the proficiencies and outcomes of their student's programme.

There are a number of expectations of practice supervision outlined by the NMC (2018c), along with the roles and responsibilities and information on the practice supervisor's contribution to assessment and progression.

Any support, training and education of supervisors needs to address these categories.

ACTIVITY 2.1

Can I be a practice supervisor?

Example 1: I completed a Preparation for Mentorship Module that complied with the Supporting, Learning and Assessment standards NMC (2008). Do I need to attend other training to meet the standards for this new role?

Answer: Having completed this programme you can be a practice supervisor for students. It is important to note that you will need to be up to date and proficient in current practice in your placement area. Access practice supervisor updates to reinforce the changes to the NMC Standards.

These will either be provided by your workplace or the AEIs that supply you with students.

Example 2: I am a newly qualified registered nurse and I would really like to contribute to the supervision of student nurses. What training do I need to attend?

Answer: Newly qualified nurses are permitted to be practice supervisors (NMC, 2018c). Your AEI and your practice placement area will offer training on how to be a practice supervisor to prepare you for this role.

As a practice supervisor there are many responsibilities and as a registrant you must follow your code of practice when supporting a student in practice. The next box summarises these.

_____ WHAT IS EXPECTED OF ME AS A _____ PRACTICE SUPERVISOR?

I have recently been assigned to be a practice supervisor for a Year 1 Trainee Nursing Associate. I have attended my local AEI study period to become a practice supervisor. What is expected of me?

- I need to act as a role model for my student delivering safe and effective practice according to my code of conduct.
- I need to identify my scope of practice in relation to the proficiencies that the student needs to meet for their programme.
- I need to supervise my student, facilitate their learning in a supportive manner.
- I will provide my student with constructive feedback on their performance and progress.
- I will be required to provide feedback on whether or not conduct and proficiencies have been met – this could be really difficult. (See Chapter 4 for more information on giving feedback).
- I may be responsible for putting an action plan in place to improve student performance – but I can always seek support from the practice assessor.

(Continued)

- I need to keep up to date and be current in my practice related to the skills and proficiencies that my student needs to achieve.
- I should feel supported and seek assistance to enable me to be a practice supervisor.
- I need to decide what level of continued support is needed for my student. If I am not available I need to arrange another supervisor to support my student – this will be useful when the student needs to visit other departments.
- I have a responsibility to record and document my student's achievements in their placement documentation related to their conduct, professional behaviour and proficiency.
- I need to liaise with colleagues, the practice assessor and the academic assessor on my observations and documentations on my student.
- My opinion is essential in the assessment of my student.
- I must always raise any concerns that I have about my student in relation to conduct and competence.

What are the general expectations in practice? Prior to the student being allocated a number of factors will have been addressed by the education team of the institution and the AEI: please see Part 2 Standards for student supervision and assessment section 2 (NMC 2018c).

The role of the practice assessor

All students on an NMC approved programme will be assigned a nominated practice assessor for each practice placement or for a series of placements. The practice assessor must be a registered nurse, midwife, nursing associate or specialist community public health nurse with appropriate equivalent experience for the student's field of practice.

Both the practice assessor and the academic assessor have responsibilities related to the assessment process. As a registered professional, when you are making decisions relating to a student performance you need to have some accountability that this individual is meeting the required competencies related to the assessment. Practice and academic assessors are the gatekeepers to the NMC register and must ensure that students meet the proficiencies and competencies to an acceptable level prior to going forward to become registered nurses or midwives. Both practice assessor and academic assessor will need to work closely throughout a student's placement in order to evaluate and recommend the student for progression for each part of the programme. This must be in line with the programme standards as well as the relevant local and national policies. As with the practice assessor role, it is up to the AEI and the placement partners to decide on how best to prepare individuals for the role and they will base this on previous formal education or experience. Public protection must be upheld at all times and therefore evidence will need to be made available to the NMC to demonstrate that correct procedures are followed, maintaining a thorough record of the education and preparation academic assessors receive. It is essential that practice assessors meet the NMC Standards (2018c) related to supervision and assessment.

Preparation to be a practice assessor

Practice partners and AEIs need to jointly support practice assessors. Preparation of practice assessors must include ongoing support to prepare for, reflect on and develop their role. As part of their preparation practice assessors must also have an understanding of what the student is expected to achieve through proficiencies and programme outcomes. As a new practice assessor you will need to attend training in preparation for the role of assessing students in your practice area. It is essential, as a new practice assessor without any previous formal training, that you have undertaken the role of the practice supervisor. Advice regarding how much experience you require as a practice supervisor before you can progress to be a practice assessor will be provided in your local area in partnership with your AEI. This will depend on your experience. Please refer to the information earlier in relation to preparing to be a practice supervisor for what is required at that level.

ACTIVITY 2.2

Can I be a practice assessor?

Example 1: I completed a Preparation for Mentorship Module that complied with the Supporting, Learning and Assessment standards (NMC, 2008); do I need to attend other training to meet the standards for this new role?

(Continued)

Answer: Having completed this programme you will be eligible to be a practice assessor for students. Your local education teams in collaboration with the AEI will provide updates. It is important to note that you will need to be up to date and proficient in current practice in your work area but also aware of the changes in the new education curriculum relating to the current NMC Standards.

Example 2: I have been a registered nurse for seven years and have always wanted to be a mentor. What I do I have to do now to become a practice assessor?

Answer: You will need to undertake preparation to become a practice assessor if you have not previously completed a mentorship training course. AEIs and placement areas are working together to provide this training – check your local area for information.

The following scenario sets out what is expected of a practice assessor.

SCENARIO: WHAT IS EXPECTED OF ME AS A PRACTICE ASSESSOR?

I have been assigned as a practice assessor for a Year 2 Student Nurse in your placement area. I was a mentor under the previous NMC (2008) standards and I have attended my local AEI study period to convert to a practice assessor. What is expected of me?

- I must complete the student's final assessment documentation in the practice area to confirm achievement of proficiencies and programme outcomes for practice learning.
- All of my decisions are based on the information that I have received through sought feedback from the student's practice supervisors.
- Using the information available to me and my own observations of the student, including conduct, proficiency, achievement, student records, student reflections and any other resources, I must record an objective evidence-based assessment.

- My assessments of the student must be evidence-based, objective and fair. It is essential that I consider different learning styles, cultural backgrounds and communication styles in my assessment.
- I must escalate any concerns that I have if I do not believe previous assessments have been fair, due to evidence being unreliable or if it appears that due process was not followed.
- I am responsible for maintaining current relevant knowledge and expertise related to the NMC proficiencies and programme outcomes that I will be assessing.
- I will work closely with the nominated academic assessor to evaluate the student's performance and recommendation for progression for each part of the programme.
- I need to ensure that I have had sufficient opportunities to observe my student during their placement in order to complete my role in relation to assessment and progression.
- I am aware that assessment is a continuous process so I need to keep up to date with how my student is performing and achieving their proficiencies during their placement. This is not only for the student's progress but to ensure that supervision of the student has been fair and consistent.
- It is important that I am aware of the student's learning and achievement in their university work in addition to their practice.
- I need to ensure that there is communication with the nominated academic assessor for the relevant points in the programme structure and student progression (this will be advised through the AEI).
- I cannot be a practice supervisor, practice assessor or an academic assessor for the same student.
- As a registered nurse/midwife/nursing associate I have a responsibility to protect the public so I must escalate any concerns I have in accordance with NMC, AEI and local policy.
- It is my responsibility to be aware of whether or not my student is meeting the expected outcomes for this placement. I need to work collaboratively with the practice supervisor if action plans are not being achieved.
- If I have any problems or issues concerning achievement, progression and/or patient safety I need to contact the academic assessor. This may lead to fitness to practise procedures at the AEI.

(Continued)

- At the end of placement I need to ensure that I hand over the assessment responsibility to the next practice assessor, having completed the student's practice learning documents with all relevant information. I will follow any process of handover outlined by the AEIs for the next practice assessor.
- I will seek support if required and attend any training updates for this role to keep current on the proficiencies related to the student's programme.

What are the general expectations in practice?

Prior to the student being allocated there will have been a number of factors addressed by the education team of the institution and the AEI: please see Part 2 Standards for student supervision and assessment section 2 (NMC, 2018c).

The role of the academic assessor

This individual will collate and confirm student achievement of proficiencies and programme outcomes in the academic setting. They will also work closely with the practice assessor to evaluate and recommend the student for progression for each part of the programme. There is an expectation that the academic assessor will enable scheduled communication and collaboration with practice assessors and any other academic assessors involved in the student's progression.

Preparation of the academic assessor

It is widely accepted that the academic assessor will be a university lecturer employed by your associated AEI. It will not always be appropriate or feasible that the academic assessor is your link lecturer/tutor. This is due to a number of factors which include availability and/or being an academic assessor for the same student on a previous placement. It is not essential that the academic assessor is a university lecturer; many placement areas have senior staff within education roles and it is an established practice to prepare these staff to become academic assessors in line with the NMC guidance and in collaboration with the AEI. The academic assessor must hold the relevant qualifications or be working towards achievement of these as required by the

AEI and must demonstrate that they meet the minimum requirements for the role (NMC, 2018c).

All assessments throughout the student's programme should be undertaken with the same rigour, standard and professionalism from their first through to their final placement, prior to qualification. Under the previous system of supporting and learning assessment in practice (NMC 2008), the status of 'sign-off mentor' was viewed as a significant responsibility for the mentor, with additional criteria needing to be met. Under the new system, an assessor with suitable preparation, experience and support should be able to accurately judge a student's suitability to complete their current placement and their final placement. There is no requirement now for a sign-off mentor in the new standards for education (NMC, 2018a).

In preparing to be a practice assessor it is important that aspects of communication, teaching/learning and assessment skills are included in the training materials. Some of the content for this preparation should be conducted in a classroom-based setting where discussion and role play can be facilitated to demonstrate understanding. Alongside this, some theoretical knowledge can be delivered through online learning materials, books and journals.

Resources available

By far, the most valuable resource that any educator would wish for is (protected) time. In the previous system under the NMC (2008), supporting learning and assessing in the clinical practice, it was recommended that student mentors had ten days protected to complete their learning on a preparation for mentorship module approved by the NMC. Many studies indicated that these student mentors did not receive this protected time while studying and, consequently, once qualified to support students in the clinical area there was no specific allocated time for mentors and their students. The role of sign-off mentor for final placement assessment and midwifery assessment also required the 'mentor' to have protected time. Evidence shows that this time was not readily available to sign-off mentors. For the current standards NMC (2018a) there are no specified hours or dedicated time suggested to supervise and assess students. As a supervisor and an assessor it is recommended that you identify the time required to spend with your learner dependent on their learning needs and negotiate this time with your manager. Practice assessment documents require time and patience to complete and these documents are the evidence that supervision and assessment have taken place. It is vital to ensure sufficient time has been negotiated to be able to deliver the actual teaching, learning and assessment needed to take students successfully through their placement, not forgetting the completion of the student's placement documentation. Walsh (2014) outlines how staff in the placement area are one of the most valuable resources available to students. As a practice supervisor or as a practice assessor, include your team and the extended interdisciplinary team in your facilitation of your student's learning.

ACTIVITY 2.3

Reflection on your practice area

How does your practice area provide time for supervisors to be with their learners?

What will you do to ensure that you have protected time with your student learner?

The NMC (2018a, 2018b, 2018c) has produced standards in three parts to address the new education standards for pre-registration student nurses. In addition to these documents, which can be downloaded from their website, there are additional explanatory documents available. This website should be accessed on a regular basis to review these documents in relation to nurse education (www.nmc.org.uk/standards).

Utilising student feedback to enhance the educators' and assessors' development

As practice supervisors, practice assessors and academic assessors, providing students and learners with feedback is an essential part of the role. Please see Chapter 4 for information related to providing feedback.

In this chapter the focus is on how the educators and assessors utilise their student's feedback on their supervising and assessing skills. Without this feedback how are you expected to improve and enhance your own development? Evaluation of learning during and at the end of a practice placement may cover many aspects of the student's learning, however it is important that the student's feedback is collated and acted upon. Listening to your student and gaining their feedback is paramount in gaining their trust and consolidating their role in the team. You may not always be in a position to address some of the issues raised by students but listening and escalating when necessary enhances the student trust in you. Elcock and Sharples (2011) recommend potential areas for evaluation:

- The student's experience while on placement
- The quality of the placement as a learning environment
- Your own experiences as a practice supervisor and/or practice assessor
- Your role as a practice supervisor and/or assessor.

All of the above are an excellent way to evaluate the whole experience of supervision and assessment. The final two relating to you, your experiences and your role, may be useful for professional development, your appraisal and your NMC revalidation. Using a reflective model or framework will assist you to identify areas of development on a personal level. Gibbs (1988) remains a popular reflective model for nurses due to the stages that assist you to work through your reflection. Use Gibbs' stages outlined here to assist you to reflect.

1. Describe the experience or activity in objective detail.
2. Discuss and explore any feelings that you experienced at the time of the experience.
3. Evaluate the experience. What happened? What was good and what was bad about the experience? Were there any contributing factors?
4. Analyse the experience: what can you learn from it?
5. Conclusion: is there anything you could have done differently? If you could change the situation, what would you do now?
6. Action place: how and what could you do differently in the future?

With regards to the student's evaluation you may choose to do this in a number of formats. During assessments it is recommended that you receive verbal feedback from your student in a reciprocal discussion which you need to address in the moment. Following reflection on this feedback you can learn and introduce changes based on your own experiences. At the end of a placement it is advisable that students complete an evaluation form based on their experiences during their time with you. Asking the students to complete this form following their final assessment may promote a more honest response to the questions on the form. Final assessments should not include any surprises related to student performance and grading, therefore a student should not be afraid of failing without due discussion. Students remain fearful that if they provide honest feedback, be it positive or negative, it will affect their final assessment.

Completing an evaluation form will assist the supervisors and assessors in a placement area and it will also help to contribute to education audits and Care Quality Commission (CQC) visits. Comments can contribute to ways of improving the learning environment.

CHAPTER SUMMARY

In this chapter we have:

- Discussed the role of the educator
- Discussed the role of the supervisor
- Discussed the role of the assessor
- Discussed the role of the academic assessor
- Suggested ideas regarding the resources available to educators and assessors for supporting learners in practice
- Promoted the use of reflection to learn from student feedback to enhance the educator's and assessor's development in practice.

3

UNDERSTANDING THE CURRICULUM AND SUPPORTING STUDENTS THROUGH ASSESSMENT

STANDARD 5

Curricula and assessment

S5.1 Curricula and assessments are developed, implemented and reviewed to ensure that students achieve the learning outcomes and NMC proficiencies for their approved programme (NMC, 2018a).

AIMS OF THIS CHAPTER

- To understand the nature of the curricula and how to support students through their academic course
- To understand assessment and the importance of reliability and validity within the assessment process
- To understand the role of the practice and academic assessor in this process
- To understand accountability and its importance in assessment.

Introduction

The curricula are components we study to be a registered nurse or other healthcare professional. It is important that the curriculum addresses and teaches components that are relevant to the expected qualification. For example, we don't teach nurses how to perform abdominal surgery because they will never do this as part of their professional role. The curriculum is developed over three years to progress the student through basic to complex material; they will learn anatomy and physiology in the first year which will aid learning of pharmacology in the third year.

Assessment allows us to measure the progress of students through various stages of training, so that successful students can move on to further training and learning. We need student nurses to be assessed theoretically and clinically to ensure that they have the knowledge base, clinical skills and professional attitude to successfully join the nursing register.

Curricula

A new curriculum is created whenever an educational institution deems that a new programme or a new module is required. The appropriate qualified personnel will then be involved in the design, development and delivery of this new curriculum. In the case of student nurses and other healthcare practitioners, they will be undertaking a programme approved by the NMC or another regulatory body. For nursing curricula, the NMC (2018a) quality assurance states that the standards for nurse education and the education providers must meet the expected criteria and be validated prior to implementation. This is known as conjoint validation where the NMC, the education provider and other stakeholders are equal partners in the entire validation process (Hughes and Quinn, 2013). As nursing is a graduate-level profession, the programme design must also meet the education provider's validation criteria.

In order to meet the NMC proficiencies for a new programme curriculum it is essential that the development of the course work involves a variety of partners. Practice partners, current student nurses, service users, nursing academics and support staff such as librarians all play an essential role in the development of a new curriculum. Clinical staff and practice partners are invited to participate in the formulation of a new curriculum as a quality assurance measure. Good collaboration with practice partners influences the relationship and helps to bridge the theory to practice gap.

Theory and practice need to be identified and introduced in increasing levels of complexity, structured in a way that allows students to manage their learning. For example, the skill and competence of taking and recording vital signs is built upon incrementally over three years. A Year 1 student will be expected to perform the skill proficiently and accurately. They must report their findings in the patient records and inform their senior or their practice supervisor of the results which may result in escalation of patient care. The student's knowledge and understanding of the results and their interpretation of the results will improve with experience and therefore by Year 3 of their programme their practice should have improved. University lectures will cover additional information on physiology and the scientific knowledge related to interpreting clinical findings. If you are their practice supervisor you will be implementing the practice element of the curriculum in your daily supervision and education of your student/learner. The recording of vital signs is an excellent example of how you need to interpret your support for the students you are supervising and assessing. Consider all of the competencies that the student needs to achieve in your practice placement, ranging from communication to wound care, medicine rounds to the dying patient. You need to maintain and further develop your knowledge on these skills and competencies as part of your registration and remain current on relevant evidence-based practice (NMC, 2018e).

As a student progresses through each part of their programme their knowledge and skills will develop further en route to becoming a registered professional. Linking theoretical knowledge from academic practice to clinical practice is essential for this progression and development. As a practice supervisor or assessor you will be ideally placed to help facilitate this learning for your student. By encouraging students to make these links you can be instrumental in putting the curriculum into practice on an everyday basis. All of your experience is vital when preparing the future healthcare professionals, with the ultimate aim of protecting the public (NMC, 2018e). You are protecting the public by ensuring that students are following their curriculum, practising with and being assessed by registered professionals with a current and relevant evidence base.

Using your knowledge and expertise as a practice supervisor or a practice assessor you could consider developing your teaching skills further by participating in the delivery of the academic element of the student's programme at the AEI. Clinical staff are a valuable asset to the AEI on many levels and there could be opportunities to contribute directly within the classroom setting. Just like clinical supervisors and assessors, all lecturers have a professional responsibility to remain up to date with practice. However, the students often appreciate and are sometimes more engaged when staff from practice contribute to lectures in person. This also helps to strengthen further the relationship between AEIs and practice providers.

ACTIVITY 3.1

Reflection on participating in curricula delivery

Spend a few moments thinking about ways you could participate in the delivery of curricula.

To help you to understand the process involved with curriculum planning and design it is suggested that you consider a number of teaching sessions for your own area of expertise and devise a plan to deliver these to your learners. For example, setting up a mini-course for a learner in your operating department could take the form of teaching sessions on:

1. Scrubbing, gowning and gloving in the theatre environment
2. Effective and efficient circulating/scouting in the operating theatre
3. How to lay an instrument trolley while scrubbed in the operating theatre
4. Techniques required when running/managing an operating list in theatre.

ACTIVITY 3.2

Developing a mini-course

Work through the following questions to help you design an effective course.

What are the learning outcomes required to meet your mini-course? (Consider each teaching session individually).

What is the theory required to meet your learning outcomes? How much and when will it be taught/delivered?

What experts do you need to assist you in the delivery of your teaching sessions/mini-course?

How and where will you teach your theoretical and your practice content?

Who is eligible to undertake your mini-course?

How will you facilitate your learners in achieving their learning outcomes?

How will you assess your students?

How will you support students if they are not successful in this mini-course?

What is your time scale for completing this mini-course?

Use this activity in your own placement area to introduce teaching sessions applicable to your own requirements. By following the above criteria, you will have an experience of what it is like to set up your own course and curriculum. Your education team may wish to make your plans more formal and therefore require some in-house validation process.

Assessment

Students are continually assessed throughout their nurse training. Continual assessment takes many forms, both formative and summative. Formative assessment is carried out to check a learner's level of progress or understanding; summative assessment is conducted to gauge competency measured against an established standard or benchmark. Assessment also spans both theoretical components delivered by higher education institutes and the assessment of skills, knowledge and attitudes in clinical practice. Nursing students will be assessed against competencies and judged whether or not they are safe to practise a skill. We assess students to ensure that they have reached approved criteria, ensuring that all student nurses reach the levels of attainment expected for their level of training. In the UK this means that every qualified and registered nurse has met the standards required for nursing as set out by the Nursing and Midwifery Council.

To ensure that we assess students fairly, practice assessors should have an initial interview early in the student's placement. This could include an orientation to the clinical area but should also address the student's expectations. Communicating this clearly at the outset will mean that the student will understand what can be achieved during their time in the clinical area as well as what won't be covered at this stage. Giving clear guidance at the outset also means that students are less likely to fail, but if they do fail they cannot complain that they did not receive guidance and support. The information in the next box sets out some questions you could consider at an initial meeting.

AREAS TO CONSIDER WITH STUDENTS AT INITIAL MEETING

- What is the student hoping to cover in this placement?
- Do they have outstanding skills that they need to achieve?
- How have they got on in other placements?
- Have these been positive or negative experiences?
- What are the practice assessors' expectations of the placement?

Listen to the student's responses. What are they telling you? Are they enjoying their training? Do they have any anxieties?

Formative assessment

Formative assessment provides ongoing feedback. It helps students to understand their strengths and weaknesses, and helps assessors to focus their teaching and support on weak areas. It comes in different forms and can be conducted through a simple conversation and some well selected questions or more structured approaches like a short test or quiz.

Summative assessment

Summative assessment tests whether students have gained certain levels of knowledge and clinical skills, measured against an established benchmark. It can take different forms ranging from a written exam or an assignment to assess clinical practice.

Table 3.1 summarises some of the most common forms of formative and summative assessment.

Table 3.1   Types of assessment

Type of assessment	How it is used
Formative	Mid-way clinical assessments
	Academic feedback
	Practice exams
	Observing clinical practice and feedbacking on skills
	Drug rounds
	Questioning students on their knowledge
	Observing students' attitudes and feeding back to the student
Summative	Final exams under exam conditions
	Submitted assignments and coursework
	Assessed clinical practice

Validity

When assessing a student, it is important to consider how valid your assessment is of them. Put simply, validity is the extent to which the test measures what it is meant to measure. For example, the NMC asks that your assessment is based on working with the student: it would not be a fair or valid assessment if you passed or failed a student having worked with them for a single day. Another example would be that it is unfair to test a first year student nurse on third year student nurse learning outcomes because they would not yet have been prepared for this level of assessment. To increase the validity of your assessment you would observe a student more than once to ensure that they are continuing to practise a skill. This might be direct observation initially then indirect observation. Continuous assessment of a student is useful because you can assess them over time.

Reliability

Reliability is how consistent your assessment is: does it measure what it is designed to measure? It is important as an assessor that you are reliable in your assessment so that you consistently pass and fail students for the same clinical skills and not decide arbitrarily to pass a student on a whim or because you like them.

How do we assess students?

- Through formative and summative exams and assignments
- Through observation of their clinical practice including their attitudes to patients
- Through questioning
- Through discussion with the practice supervisor and assessor and the academic assessor.

The NMC have previously said that students should be supervised in the practice setting for at least 40 per cent of their clinical placement by their practice assessor (NMC, 2006, 2008).

Under the new system the NMC guidance is contained in Realising Professionalism: Standards for Education and Training. Part 2: Standards for Student Supervision and Assessment does not stipulate a specific amount of time but says:

> the decision on the level of supervision provided for students should be based on the needs of the individual student. The level of supervision can decrease with the student's increasing proficiency and confidence. (NMC, 2018b: 4)

Judgement is therefore required about how much supervision students require. Although there are no longer strict levels specified by the NMC (i.e. 40 per cent of time) students will still need strong levels of initial supervision to allow you to build up a picture of their confidence and proficiency. If the student demonstrates good performance this may mean they can work unsupervised for more of the time. On the other hand, if they are struggling you may deem it necessary for them to spend more than 40 per cent of their time under supervision.

Failing students

Kathleen Duffy's work on 'Failing to fail' students provides practice assessors with important insights into their role and the difficulties of failing students. She found that assessors were more likely to pass a student as competent even when there were doubts about the student nurse's clinical skills. Her research found that weak students often had a history of problems in clinical practice and were more likely to be passed than failed. Duffy found that nurses' assessors were more likely to be influenced by a student's personal problems and would allow this to influence their decisions, allowing students to progress onto the next part of their training. She argued that:

> When mentors decide to give the students the 'benefit of the doubt' it appears that they are not usually aware of the possible consequences of their actions i.e. that these students often progress in the programme without their problems being adequately addressed. (Duffy, 2003: 70)

It is important to identify failing students at the earliest opportunity so that action can be taken to support and help them succeed. Where despite support and interventions a student is still unable to meet the required standards, the outcome would be a fail. It is important to act decisively when students are failing to give them the best chance of reaching a good outcome. Delaying a decision to intervene or fail a student is not in anyone's best interest. Failing a student at the end of the programme when this should have been done earlier wastes student's time and means that they have incurred higher levels of financial debt. It is important to address any issues early and support students to avoid this if possible, but you should support them through failing as well.

How to cope with failing students

Students who are failing should not get to the end of a placement and then find this out. They should have had an introductory and formative assessment to highlight areas in which they are not doing well and how to improve in them. An action plan may need to be devised to help the student become competent. This is an excellent tool as it will show a student where they need to improve and what to do, and the practice assessor, supervisor and academic assessor will need to be involved in the action plan and help support the student. These actions should mean that the student who is about to fail is aware that this is likely to happen because they have not met the action plan. The action plan also helps the assessors to clearly document areas in which the student is failing.

ACTIVITY 3.3

Reflection on failure

Have you ever failed something? How did it feel? How were you told?

Everyone at some point in their lives fails something. It may seem like a disaster at the time. If you have failed how did you find out? Would you have done it differently in their shoes? What was good or bad about the way you were told?

How to tell a student they are failing their placement

- Consider the emotional issues for you and the student – how will they respond?
- Discuss your reasons with the academic assessor – they are there to support you and the student.
- Discuss the situation with your manager so that time can be allocated to discuss the situation.
- Record why you are failing the student and the reasons behind this.
- Meet with the student privately to break the news and explain why.
- Deal with the student's response. They may be upset or angry.
- Be prepared for how you feel – this is stressful.

This scenario illustrates a failing student.

———————————— SCENARIO ————————————

Unprofessional behaviour

Jay is a first year student nurse. His assessor has told him that he needs to address his unprofessional behaviour. Jay has missed several days of his clinical placement and not informed the ward. He has arrived late for shifts. His practice assessor Rosie has contacted the academic assessor, Carol, and discussed the situation with her. Rosie has offered Jay more time to make up the missed sessions, but he has missed more due to sickness.

Carol has asked to meet Jay, but he has missed this session as well. Jay has missed so much time he cannot make it up in this placement. Jay has been asked for proof of sickness which he has not supplied. He has been offered counselling services but has declined. Carol and Rosie have spoken to him about his unprofessional attitude because he has failed to contact staff when he is sick. Rosie fails Jay at the end of the placement, Jay is very angry, but Rosie points out she has not worked with him enough to assess him. He will be offered another placement for reassessment. Jay complains to the university about his placement. However this is not upheld as all the documentation shows that he has been offered help and support and records his lack of communication with the team.

Rosie has kept notes of all the contact she has had with Jay, and with her manager and Carol. Carol has also kept this information.

Jay's attitude has not changed, and his lack of communication and professionalism is why he has failed this placement. However, he has another attempt to turn things around. The difficulty with this scenario is that, because Jay is off sick so much, it is difficult to talk to him about his professionalism. However, we need nurses to inform us when they are off sick so that we can organise staff to look after patients, so this is a professional issue we need Jay to understand.

The next scenario illustrates another student who is failing.

———————————— SCENARIO ————————————

Failing a summative assessment

Esther is a post-registered nurse who is undertaking a module with clinical placements on prescribing. Esther is quite quiet in class but answers questions correctly when asked. Her practice assessor, Mary, has contacted the module leader saying they are concerned about Esther. Esther has been working with Mary for three weeks. The module leader meets with Mary and discusses her concerns.

Mary is concerned that Esther lacks knowledge on pharmacology. The module leader addresses the content of the module and the assessments. Esther has failed the practice exam paper and she discusses the

(Continued)

areas in which Esther has not done well. She has already done this with Esther and is surprised that Esther has not discussed this with Mary.

Esther fails the pharmacology exam; the module leader organises to meet with Mary and Esther to review how she has got on. Esther says she is confident that she can pass her exam a second time. This will be her last opportunity as she is only given two chances to pass. The module leader reminds her of online resources available to help her. The module leader asks Esther what pharmacology books she is using to help revise. Esther has no pharmacology books and has not accessed any from the library. The module leader warns her that she was advised at the onset of the course and throughout the course to read other sources of information to aid learning.

Esther retakes the exam for the second and final time and fails. The module leader notifies the practice assessor and Esther. The practice assessor is warned that Esther has failed the course, but Mary notes that Esther's lack of knowledge meant she would have failed the clinical component too.

The module leader meets with Esther to discuss the situation. They meet privately. Esther is upset and asks if she can have another go. The module leader is firm – she has had two attempts and there are no exten-uating circumstances – but she gives Esther time and listens to her anger. Esther realises she left it too late to start working for the exam. Esther can reapply to do the course, but she will need to show the module leader what she would do differently.

Notes about this scenario

Throughout the course the module leader has given clear guidance about the passing and failing of the assessment. This is also docu-mented in the module handbooks. Esther has been given online resources to access to help revision but has also had days with teach-ing on all theory. The practice assessor has had sessions with the module leader, so they are clear about the assessment components. Mary has given one-to-one support on helping to translate theory to practice. If these areas had not been covered comprehensively Esther could have had the potential for a complaint. However, all the areas have been covered and all the other students in the class have passed first time. If a high proportion of students had failed, then the course material and teaching would need to be reviewed.

If Esther's assessor or module leader had been persuaded to pass her then an unsafe nurse would be passed as deemed competent to prescribe. This would put patients at risk and illustrates why it is a huge responsibility to pass or fail a student.

Accountability within student assessment

Practice and academic assessors are accountable for every decision they take when judging whether to pass a student nurse as competent and they need to be aware of the consequences of failing to fail an unsuitable student. Failing to fail a student may result in an incompetent student being registered as a nurse and put patients in danger. The Nursing and Midwifery Council may ask you to explain why you have passed a student who has been found to be unsafe to practise.

ACTIVITY 3.4

Reflection on fitness to practise

Have you ever looked at the NMC website detailing cases where nurses have lost their nursing registration? Go to the NMC website (www.nmc.org.uk) and briefly read through some examples.

What common issues can you identify in the cases where nurses are investigated by the Nursing and Midwifery Council?

If a nurse is taken off the NMC register, then they can no longer work as a nurse or midwife. Before striking a nurse off the NMC register the panel considers the following three questions (NMC, 2018f):

- Do the regulatory concerns about the nurse or midwife raise fundamental questions about their professionalism?
- Can public confidence in nurses and midwives be maintained if the nurse or midwife is not removed from the register?
- Is striking-off the only sanction which will be sufficient to protect patients, members of the public or maintain professional standards?

The NMC considers allegations about fraudulent or incorrect entry on the register, misconduct, lack of competence, criminal convictions and cautions, health, not having the necessary knowledge of English (for example, drug errors or poor handover), determinations by other health or social organisations. All these areas could be considered as serious professional allegations. Health is usually dealt with by managers, but nurses who show no insight into their physical or mental health are a concern if there is a risk to the public (NMC, 2018f). When failing a student, it is important to remember that if you pass them, they could be looking after you or a member of your family. Would you consider them safe to do this? It is hard to fail someone, but if you pass someone who is not safe to practise you may feel much worse.

CHAPTER SUMMARY

In this chapter we have:

- Looked at the concept of curricula – quality assurance states the standards demanded of nurse education; the education providers must meet these criteria and be validated prior to their implementation
- Discussed how clinical practice plays an important role in helping students meet the curriculum
- Looked at the different forms of assessment: through formative and summative examination and assignments, observation of clinical practice, questioning, discussion with practice supervisor and assessor and the academic assessor
- Considered the notion of 'failing to fail' as articulated by Kathleen Duffy which shows us that weak students often have a history of problems in clinical practice and were more likely to be passed than failed
- Discussed strategies for managing failure
- Described accountability as the professional responsibility nurses have to their patients and colleagues.

4

ENABLING AN EFFECTIVE LEARNING CULTURE

STANDARD 1

Learning culture

S1.1   Learning culture prioritises the safety of people including carers, students and educators, and enables the values of *The Code* to be upheld.

S1.2   Education and training is valued in all learning environments.

> ## AIMS OF THIS CHAPTER
>
> - To understand what makes a positive learning culture
> - To understand what makes a learning culture 'toxic'
> - To understand our responsibilities to raise concerns
> - To understand how we collaborate to create a learning culture.

Introduction

The way we learn is influenced by previous experiences of learning and teaching. These experiences may be positive, but they may also be negative. Positive experiences encourage learning and help make the subject area memorable.

They encourage us to think and develop. Negative experiences may make us believe we cannot do something and these can become self-fulfilling prophecies. Due to a lack of confidence we then seek to avoid that area.

ACTIVITY 4.1

Reflection on learning experiences

Try to remember your learning experiences at school. Was there anyone who supported you or taught you something you remember? What was good about this experience? Did you have any experiences that were not positive? Why was this not a valuable experience?

Have these experiences influenced the way you learn now?

Good experiences of learning are often associated with words such as supportive, encouraging, accepting, patience, enjoyable, listened, understanding. Whilst negative experiences can provoke feelings or memories of being bullied, belittled, feeling stupid.

Accountability and raising concerns

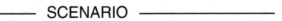 SCENARIO

A toxic learning culture

Layla is working in theatres and learning to scrub. This is not the first time she has scrubbed but she is nervous and feels the pressure to get this role right. The surgeon is renowned for being exacting and shouting at staff. The surgeon shouts at her, requesting instruments. The more she is shouted at to be quick the more nervous she becomes and the more mistakes she makes.

Layla feels humiliated and bullied. She does not feel she can speak up against this experienced doctor and feels it would be unprofessional to do so. No one speaks up for her in the theatre or speaks to her afterwards, so she feels she must be awful as a scrub nurse. Layla puts up with the shouting but decides that she won't work in this area in the future.

As educators what do you think about this scenario? Is it appropriate for a health professional to speak to another in this way? What would you do in this situation?

Let's think about how you might go about addressing a scenario like this. First, it is important to speak to the student afterwards and make sure she is feeling OK. It may be appropriate to speak to the surgeon prior to future operations to remind them they have a learner present. But the surgeon's behaviour is intimidating, and this should be addressed. An initial step would be to report the surgeon's behaviour to the nurse in charge. Often people put up with bad behaviour from others, so the person is likely to continue behaving in this way for long periods of time. This surgeon's behaviour is unprofessional, but the nurse feels it is not appropriate to speak up at the time as it could affect patient care. By staying quiet, however, the nurse is colluding with the bad behaviour. Part of the nurse's role is accountability, and this means speaking up and raising concerns and the nurse can do this after the event and not affect patient care. The nurse's practice assessor should also raise concern about the surgeon's behaviour by speaking to the nurse in charge. This scenario is an example of a toxic environment where staff feel unable to speak up against a colleague's unprofessional behaviour.

The NMC's *Code: Professional Standards of Practice and Behaviour for Nurses, Midwives and Nursing Associates* (2018e) sets clear expectations and demands of the profession, one of which is prioritising people. It asks that as nurses and midwives we 'Treat people as individuals and uphold their dignity'. It continues to say that we should 'work in partnership with people to make sure [we] deliver care effectively' (NMC, 2018: 4) and it is only by speaking up that this can be achieved. Layla should be supported by the practice assessor or practice supervisor to achieve this. However, if Layla is not supported by her nominated practice assessor, she can access support from her nominated academic assessor or the clinical link tutor. If Layla finds these assessors unsupportive then she can speak to her programme leader. These assessors and tutors are registered nurses and have a duty of care to Layla and to patients, so their roles require them to respond to Layla. If Layla is a registered nurse, then she should discuss the surgeon's behaviour with the ward manager. It is important that she does raise the issue because his behaviour could affect patient care. All health professionals work to codes of professional behaviour; the surgeon will work to the General Medical Council's *Good Medical Practice* which discusses working collaboratively with colleagues and says, 'you must treat colleagues fairly and with respect' (2013: 14). So the surgeon here is in breach of his code of professional behaviour. The surgeon's behaviour can be addressed by the nurse's practice assessor speaking directly to him, but this may be challenging to do, particularly if there is a difference in their levels of seniority, and it is likely to be influenced by the relationship of the doctor and the practice assessor. If this approach is difficult or inadequate then the practice assessor's line manager should be approached who could address the situation by talking to the surgeon's line manager. This is important because it means that patterns of poor behaviour are recorded. If this has happened before an action plan can be devised to work with the surgeon and address their behaviour.

Following the inquiry into patient care at Mid-Staffordshire Hospital a lack of care and compassion by nurses was noted. However Mid-Staffordshire Hospital was found to have had large staff shortages (Gillen, 2013), and whilst there is no argument that the care at Mid Staffordshire Hospital was poor, Paley (2014) argues that the Mid-Staffordshire Hospital incidents did not happen because of a lack of compassion and care, as reported in the media, but as a result of a staff stressed through shortages and unsustainable workload. This resulted in nurses being unable to show compassion and care, through social cognition and the unrealistic expectations placed upon them. The nursing director of Mid-Staffordshire NHS Foundation Trust gave evidence at the NMC hearing. Ms Harry said for the 29 charges against her that she expected nurses to solve issues around bed management and not rely on her. She was slated for reducing nurses to tears and for staff shortages, which saw one nurse responsible for 17 patients (Gillen, 2013). Following this inquiry, the emphasis both within the 'The Code' and in the 'Duty of Candour' puts the responsibility on the individual to speak up and not on the manager or the service (DOH, 2014). So, it is important for nurses to speak up about poor care and unprofessional behaviour to maintain their registration as nurses and protect patients. Other health professionals have similar duties to report under their professional qualification.

Helen Donnelly raised many concerns about the standards and staffing levels in the emergency department of Mid-Staffordshire Foundation Trust (Calkin, 2011). She reported the culture of fear and the massaging of waiting times to meet the four-hour target. She was threatened by staff for reporting her concerns and spoke at the inquiry into Mid-Staffordshire Foundation Trust. However, her persistence and integrity have been recognised as she was appointed the ambassador for cultural change and she has been awarded an OBE. If like Helen Donnelly there are patterns of poor care that you have raised with a manager that have not been resolved, you should contact the Freedom To Speak Up Guardians (FTSUGs) (NHS Improvement, 2018).

EXAMPLES OF TOXIC LEARNING CULTURE

- Shortage of staff
- Bullying from colleagues or managers
- Belittling of staff by colleagues or managers
- Discrimination or favouritism of a member of the team
- Management which is unavailable or unseen
- Lack of recognition of staff work in the clinical area
- Lack of time to have lunch break or an expectation that staff will work beyond finish time
- Lack of acknowledgement of skills and knowledge from prior experience
- Lack of induction: 'dropping people in at the deep end'
- Poor communication, not listening to health professionals within the work environment
- Lack of development of health professional careers
- Lack of interest in support or mentoring students
- Expectation that staff will work beyond their competence
- Frequent turnover of staff
- Unprofessional behaviour – staff turning up late or being rude to patients or staff.

These examples equal a dysfunctional workplace.

Discrimination and working environments

Another area which creates a toxic work environment is discrimination and this has the potential to negatively affect the learning culture that students will be experiencing. For instance, the Stonewall report (Somerville, 2015) explores the treatment of LGBT people within health and social care services and provides grim reading on the culture many of us work in. Of the 3,100 health and social care workers asked about their experiences relating to lesbian, gay, bisexual and trans (LGBT) issues:

- 24 per cent of patient-facing staff have heard their colleagues making negative comments about LGBT people.
- 26 per cent of LGBT staff have personally experienced bullying in the last five years because of their sexuality (Somerville, 2015).
- 16 per cent (one in six) of patient-facing staff did not feel sufficiently confident to challenge discriminating remarks heard about LGBT people (Somerville, 2015).

This report was examining just one aspect of prejudice but it raises the broader question of how to tackle discrimination within the healthcare workplace. The answer is by treating everyone with respect and increasing our awareness and understanding of different communities and minority groups. We can also educate nurses about diversity during their undergraduate nursing programme so health professionals treat people holistically. But we also need to speak up if we see discrimination and, as supervisors, assessors or educators, we need to encourage all health professionals to have the confidence to speak up as well. This will ensure that we create an honest and open environment.

With increasing numbers leaving the profession (Royal College of Nursing, 2017b), creating an enjoyable and supportive working environment has never been so important (Jones-Barry, 2018). The NMC conducted a survey with 4,500 nurses and midwives who had left the NMC register over the last year for reasons other than retirement. The top reasons for leaving the profession were working conditions, including staff shortages, changes in personal circumstances such as ill health and caring responsibilities, and a disillusionment with the quality of care provided to patients (NMC, 2017a).

The current high levels of attrition within the profession, and research like the Stonewall report demonstrate that conditions are often challenging. This has implications for the students coming into practice learning environments for the first time and it is important that educators and supervisors consider how best to mitigate this and provide the right conditions for effective learning to take place.

The learning environment

To ensure that students have an effective and positive experience in the learning environment it should be properly planned and organised. Prior to the student arriving, a named practice supervisor and assessor should be allocated to the student. It is good practice to try and arrange the rota so that the student works with their practice supervisor and assessor for their practice allocation. This will ensure that they have worked with the student for a sufficient amount of time to be able to accurately assess them.

Ideally, students should be sent a welcome pack with details of their placement, including things like uniform requirements (if applicable), relevant information about the clinical area and details such as whom to contact if sick. Practice based learning units within higher education institutes will be able to provide student allocation lists and students' university email addresses. You may want to send some pre-clinical area reading that is specific to the work you do.

Induction

On the first day of the placement the clinical area will need to work through any standard practices or policies that they have in place. For instance, there may be a requirement to confirm that the student has completed annual mandatory training for moving and handling, basic life support, and fire, health and safety; local guidelines may also need to be studied.

The educator will need to orientate the student to the clinical area, highlighting fire procedures and emergency procedures. This can be done in several ways: you can organise an induction day for a group of students; you could attach the student to various members of the team so that they learn how the clinical area functions. Students can find new clinical areas very overwhelming, and health professionals who are used to this area may forget how stressful it can be to enter a new environment. At the first meeting with the student the educator should discuss the student's expectations of this new clinical environment and what can be achieved during this placement. Dates should be organised for mid-point and final feedback so that the student understands the time limits they are working towards. A planned induction with support can reduce student's anxiety and stress levels and will foster a better learning environment (Emanuel, 2013). Chan's work endorses this and argues that student anxiety is reduced if clinical placements are supportive, and students feel accepted and trusted; if their contribution to patient care is recognised; and if teaching is current and opportunities to practise are given (Chan, 2004). Remember that this is your area of expertise, but your student may feel nervous or anxious about looking after children or patients who are dying, for example, so try to address any anxieties early and show them how you cope.

——————— AREAS TO COVER AT INDUCTION ———————

- Introduction to area and staff in the department
- Timetable of placement
- Uniform policy – if the student needs to wear their own clothes you should discuss appropriate clothing
- Shift patterns, meal breaks
- Fire exits and procedures and fire equipment
- Health and safety policies
- Details of student's practice assessor and supervisor and how to contact them
- Who the student should contact if they are ill
- Area of nursing the student will cover in placement
- Formative and summative interview dates
- Workbooks, resources to help the student get the most out of their environment
- Any areas the student is concerned about.

Feedback

The role of the educator is to provide a learning environment with opportunities to work with different members of the multidisciplinary team, providing supervision and a planned learning experience. Educators provide a unique opportunity to role model the professional values and behaviours of a professional nurse that are expected by the NMC, or those of another registered professional role. Educators also assess competence and provide honest and constructive feedback of the progress of the student (RCN, 2017a).

Feedback is vital to learners so that they can understand what they are getting right, and what they need to improve on. Duffy has highlighted students' dissatisfaction with the feedback they receive, saying that students find it difficult to get feedback, citing inconsistency in the amount of feedback, the type and timing of the feedback given (Duffy, 2013). Her research advocates the need for regular feedback between the educator and the student which addresses five principles. These are set out opposite.

DUFFY'S FIVE PRINCIPLES
OF FEEDBACK

- Provide realistic goals for the clinical placement and the students level of learning
- Try to understand what are the student's expectations of the feedback
- Gain feedback from other sources on the student's practice
- Act swiftly
- Be specific in the feedback you give, with illustration of examples observed.

Feedback can be given during or soon after an event, but it should also be at the beginning, in the middle and at the end of a clinical placement. It is important to allow the student your full attention and time in feedback, and this should be in a quiet area providing sufficient levels of privacy. This will encourage good levels of dialogue but will also reduce the chance of interruptions by other members of the healthcare team and patients. An example of people not giving their full attention is when friends you are socialising with frequently look at or text on their mobile phones. Do you feel OK with this or do you find this rude? Does it make you think you are maybe boring them, or that they are not interested in you? This lack of one to one attention can create these negative feelings; health professionals should not be on their personal mobile phones in the clinical area; frequent interruptions and lack of privacy can create the same feelings in students. Whilst clinical areas are very busy it is important to allow adequate time for feedback, and managers should support this. There is a clear expectation from the NMC that practice providers and HEIs work positively and collaboratively in support of nurse education. If students report negative experiences of their placements, a number of steps will be taken to understand any underlying issues and aim to improve this. At the extreme end, if clinical areas are consistently failing to provide adequate support for students their allocation of students could be stopped by higher education institutes, which will reflect on the clinical area and the hospital trust. Figures 4.1 and 4.2 provide examples of formative feedback for Tom, a second year student working on a male surgical ward.

Mid-way progress:

No problems Tom is doing well.

Areas that need developing:

Continue.

Signed: Staff nurse Jones

Figure 4.1   Example of poor formative feedback

An example of poor feedback is illustrated in Figure 4.1. It gives little information about how Tom is progressing, whilst Figure 4.2 gives constructive feedback about Tom's allocation. You can see from Figure 4.2 that other health professionals and assessors can see what the student is doing and what he needs to do to improve. There are comments about Tom's professional attitude (a key component of a nursing), and this can

---

Mid-way progress:

Tom has made a good start on the ward; he shows initiative and recognises patients' needs. He has been responsible for looking after a bay of patients, planning care and pre-operative assessment. He has followed these patients through surgery and with supervision provided post-operative care for patients following surgery after renal and prostate surgery. Tom works well within the nursing team and is a compassionate nurse. He always seeks help when needed.

Areas that need developing.

Tom needs to increase his knowledge of the pharmacology of the ward drugs particularly diuretics and hypertensive drugs. His knowledge of anatomy and physiology are good, but he needs to learn more in depth renal theory and apply this to the pharmacology. Tom is going to present to the ward team the care of a patient having a renal transplant in the last week of his placement.

Signed: Staff nurse Jones

Figure 4.2   Example of constructive formative feedback

be the area where students fail. Good nurses appear to get less feedback because they are good, however this feedback will help Tom, a good nurse, to develop further.

———————— EFFECTIVE FEEDBACK ————————

- Encourage the student to reflect on their practice. How do they think they are doing?
- Feedback from service users and other members of the multidisciplinary team should be sought.
- Feedback should be written.
- Feedback should be constructive. Negative comments should be turned into learning points and how the nurse can improve. Action plans should be created with the student so that they understand what they need to do to improve and so that competency can be assessed at the end of the placement.
- Feedback should be specific, and examples should be given to illustrate positive and negative practice.
- Feedback should be clear and objective.
- The educator should ensure the student understands the feedback. This can be done by asking open-ended questions.
- The student should be informed of any other staff who need to be involved in the feedback. This includes higher education institutes' clinical link staff.
- Finally, what is the student's feedback on the learning environment? Are they getting the learning opportunities and experiences you have organised and they requested.

Feedback may involve failing students at the end of the clinical placement and this can be distressing for both the student and the practice assessor.

If you are failing a student, this will not be a sudden decision that you have reached lightly. This will be a decision you will have considered for some time, having made every reasonable effort to help the student reach the levels of performance required. If you do find yourself in this situation you should inform the academic assessor and your manager. Write down why you are failing this student, giving the reasons and examples; what actions were taken and what were the outcomes of these actions? Also, record what the student does well. Although not necessarily pleasant, you will find this activity useful when giving the news of failure to the student, and it will help them to understand why they have failed and what they need to do to pass.

───────────── SCENARIO ─────────────

Giving feedback to a failing student

Ashley is a student nurse at the end of her first year. She has passed her clinical placements so far. However, there is very little written in her practice learning document from her previous placements.

Ashley's practice assessor Kate has found Ashley to be difficult to work with. She is not keen on doing anything and looks bored; she sometimes appears rude and is often late for her shifts. Kate has spoken to colleagues who are experiencing the same attitudes from Ashley. Kate has spoken to Ashley throughout the placement and warned her that she would fail her placement on her attitude if it did not improve. Kate has spoken to the academic supervisor.

When Kate spoke to Ashley in the formative placement, she asked Ashley if she was happy and she replied that she was unsure about a career in nursing and there were no other personal issues. Kate suggested Ashley might take up the opportunity of university counselling or see her personal tutor.

At the final interview Kate fails Ashley for the placement. Ashley is not surprised because she has been given feedback and support throughout the placement from Kate. This gives Ashley the opportunity to retake the placement and have more time to consider if nursing is for her. However, Ashley feels she wants to give up nursing and is relieved.

───────────── SCENARIO ─────────────

George is a student nurse at the end of his second year. He has passed his clinical placements and had no problems. George has been allocated to a general medical ward.

George's practice assessor is Steve who has found George a keen and intelligent student. However, one of the patients is HIV positive and Steve has noticed that George avoids looking after him. Steve asks George about this patient and George says he does not want to look after anyone who is homosexual. George holds inaccurate knowledge about HIV. Steve finds the situation difficult. He is homosexual himself and is unsure how to address these attitudes so he discusses the situation with the academic supervisor. The academic supervisor Emma meets with Steve and George. Emma discusses with George his attitudes and tells him that these do not meet the NMC's professional requirements; she suggests that George revisits these and the duty of care that nurses have to meet. Emma also gives George and Steve some literature and resources on HIV and homosexuality for George to read and discuss with Steve. An action plan is devised surrounding George's homophobic attitudes and inaccurate knowledge of HIV. George is asked to complete some written work to address these areas and submit this to Steve and Emma.

At the final interview Steve passes George; he has found that George's attitudes have changed significantly, and George is horrified that he felt as he did. George grew up in a country where homosexuality is illegal and men are imprisoned for being gay. He has grown up in a culture which has expressed different views about homosexuality and now realises that he has a duty of care to treat all patients the same. George also now holds accurate information about HIV and its transmission and treatment.

The first scenario shows that not all nurses are unhappy to fail their placement, but also highlights that lack of earlier feedback to Ashley has meant that she has not received help earlier. It is better for Ashley to fail earlier in her nursing career than get to the end of the third year, possibly having accrued more student debt and been unhappier for longer.

George's scenario shows that attitudes are important in the nursing profession and if George had not shown significant insight into his attitudes then he would have failed his clinical placement. It is important not to ignore attitudes that are discriminatory as they will increase poor nursing care. George avoided looking after homosexual patients, so this would have meant that these patients would have been neglected. It is important to remember that we all come from different backgrounds, and cultural and religious views may have created biases that nurses need to address in order to look after patients equally and compassionately. Another area that some nurses find difficult is abortion, and as a practice assessor you may have to discuss the duty of care nurses have to look after all patients.

Evaluation

Evaluation is a combined approach between the student and the educator. It gives the educator the opportunity to give final feedback but also allows the student to give feedback on their clinical experience. This feedback is important for local quality and governance monitoring such as educational audits. It can also be used for nurse educator's feedback for their revalidation with the NMC. Student evaluations should be kept for educational audits so that the auditor can review the feedback (they may also wish to meet up with a student currently in clinical placement to gain further feedback). This feedback may also be wanted for visits by the Care Quality Commission (CQC) and Nursing and Midwifery Council.

The feedback you give your student tells them how they have performed. The evaluation from the student will give you and your clinical area feedback on how you have performed. It is important to get this feedback after you have completed your feedback – students may not be honest if they think it will affect them passing their placement. Reviewing these evaluations can give you insight into how your area is seen from someone new to it. You need to look at what went well and what did not go well from the student's perspective and consider what you could do to improve their experience of your clinical area. Positive feedback should be shared with the healthcare professional team so that they are rewarded for their hard work.

CHAPTER SUMMARY

In this chapter we have:

- Explored the importance of a positive learning environment which fosters and supports the learner
- Seen how a toxic learning culture and discriminatory environment can increase disillusionment in the profession and create barriers to effective learning for students
- Discussed how feedback is an essential component of learning and needs to be relevant, constructive and specific
- Considered how evaluating the learning environment can ensure that the learner's needs are met. This feedback can be used for registered nurses' revalidation.

5

EDUCATIONAL GOVERNANCE AND QUALITY

STANDARD 2

Educational governance and quality

2.1 There are effective governance systems that ensure compliance with all legal, regulatory, professional and educational requirements, differentiating where appropriate between the devolved legislatures of the United Kingdom, with clear lines of responsibility and accountability for meeting those requirements and responding when standards are not met, in all learning environments.

2.2 All learning environments optimise safety and quality, taking account of the diverse needs of, and working in partnership with, service users, students and all other stakeholders.

AIMS OF THE CHAPTER

- To identify the quality expectations of the university and the placement area
- To offer recommendations for collaborative working
- To understand the purpose for education quality reviews/audits
- To identify the importance of including the participation of service users in nursing governance and quality

(Continued)

- Highlighting fitness to practise procedures
- To raise awareness of how to escalate concerns of practice
- To demonstrate how students are supported during placements
- To highlight the importance of documentation
- Notes on revalidation.

In this chapter there will be discussion relating to the expectations required by the education provider and the placement provider with respect to governance and quality for healthcare students. The NMC standards (2018a) will be used to guide this discussion.

Collaboration/partnership working with placement areas

One of the most tangible expectations of quality relationships with the university and the placement area is the role of the 'link lecturer/tutor'. All universities have a responsibility to have an identified member of the academic teaching team to link with practice placement areas. In addition to this role a number of other staff may be employed by the placement area who together will support students but will also be there to support you in your role as practice supervisor and/or practice assessor. Support for students will be discussed later in this chapter. Within your practice area you will most likely find access to:

Clinical placement co-ordinator: This role is usually a nurse who works in the clinical area with a responsibility to ensure that the students that are allocated to an area have an appropriate supervisor and assessor identified prior to their start date. They also have a responsibility to ensure that the staff in the area have sufficient numbers of supervisors and assessors to support student nurses on placement. This individual is employed in the placement area and works closely with one or more universities to enable suitable and safe allocations.

Link lecturer/tutor: Link tutors are university academic staff that have been allocated to clinical practice areas to support supervisors, assessors and student nurses on placement. Ideally the link tutor will have experience related to the clinical area; however this is not always feasible. This tutor is your link to the university and can help you and your colleagues solve any problems that may arise and can also assist the assessor and academic assessor with any assessment queries.

Clinical/practice educator: This educator is a nurse or other allied health professional who has undertaken training and education to become a clinical teacher and assessor. Often these educators are employed to support new staff members in addition to student nurses. They may be assigned as supervisors and assessors if they have had the appropriate training.

Academic assessor: Students will be allocated an academic assessor for each part of their programme. The academic assessor will discuss assessment with the student's practice assessor, contribute to assessment and jointly decide on progression at the appropriate times of the programme, such as progression points. See Chapter 2 for more detail on the academic assessor role.

For the success and viability of clinical learning placements it is imperative that there is a solid and supportive relationship between the education provider and the placement area. There is a variety of ways to create these relationships and a commitment from both parties to maintain a healthy status quo. With the priorities of learners being paramount for this successful relationship it is essential that both parties identify ways of meeting their respective requirements and responsibilities. Many partnerships will have regular meetings to explore ways of improving practice placements and generally to discuss and evaluate current student experience. These meetings are usually attended by the education team in your placement area; this may be the lead for clinical/practice education, it may be clinical placement facilitators, but it will usually be an individual whose role is dedicated to learning and teaching. If you are interested in understanding more about the education of clinical staff it may be worth you speaking to your line manager about attending some of these meetings; it could help you better understand the supervisor and assessor roles and may also contribute to your own career progression and development. Examples of these meetings may include:

- Supervisor/assessor support meetings
- Educational standards meetings
- Quality of clinical placement monitoring meetings
- Curriculum development meetings and more.

ACTIVITY 5.1

Involvement with curriculum development

Speak with your education lead to identify what meetings they attend with your education provider.

List the meetings attended and their purpose.

Provide examples of good practice that have improved following these meetings.

Individual universities may require educational audits or reviews to be conducted and be kept up to date in all placement areas where students are allocated. These reviews are essential to establish that the placement areas are well prepared and adequately resourced to have learners in their area. These audits/reviews contribute to the annual self-reporting to the nursing and midwifery quality assurance (QA) framework (NMC, 2018g). These audits cover a range of educational requirements for the clinical area and for the education provider, and identify quality requirements expected of each party. They include essential contact information and details on the speciality of the area which must be kept up to date. There is further information related to the learning opportunities available, potential learning outcomes, the access to the multi-professional team and the overall experience that the learner can achieve in the placement area. The review will also identify resources in relation to policy and procedure, indemnity assurances and any relevant external body reviews e.g CQC and the Office for Standards of Education, children's services and skills (Ofsted).

ACTIVITY 5.2

Education quality audit

Locate your most recent education quality review/audit.

Identify the following:

Who is responsible for completing the review?

Which other personnel may be involved in the review?

When did your last review take place?

Are all of the actions outlined in the review completed or being completed?

When is your next review due?

Are there any changes in your clinical area that may affect the next review?

How and where do the reviewers access the register of supervisors and assessors (previously mentors)?

Consider the types of evidence that can be used to meet the statements of the review.

Curriculum

Following the introduction of any new standards for education there will need to be changes implemented in the education curricula for healthcare. The standards of proficiency for registered nurses (NMC, 2018h) require all education providers to produce a new nurse education programme. This most recent version of the standards has been quite controversial with regards to the inclusion of certain new skills that, whilst beneficial from a practice perspective, are likely to pose many issues for clinical education.

The new standards of proficiency for the future nurse (NMC, 2018h) include nursing procedures required for registration. Whilst causing some controversy with the inclusion of undertaking manual evacuation of the bowels when appropriate, administering intravenous medication, venepuncture and cannulation and undertaking chest auscultation have increased the expectations of the university and also practice assessment areas to provide these experiences for student in relation to teaching and assessment. Local policies and governance groups will need to amend and approve the inclusion of these skills for student nurses to perform under supervision. It is important to add that some practice areas may not offer these skills to students due to the nature and the specialty of the area. This is relevant for many other skills that the future nurse needs to acquire; however, it is important that all supervisors and assessors are aware of the proficiencies required for these learners. For students who are unable to achieve these proficiencies in practice the university needs to have a contingency plan in place so that the students can still meet the requirements. See Chapter 3 for further information on the curriculum.

Service user involvement in curriculum development, student selection and student learning and assessment

The inclusion of service users at significant points in nurse education and the preparation of nurse education is essential to promote quality in the programme. Involvement of service users at interview and the selection process of potential student nurses not only adds to the validity of the selection process but also promotes the reality of the future of nursing to all involved in the process. In an interview situation it is often the service user who identifies reasons to reject an applicant or identifies reasons to include an applicant.

When a new programme is being written, it is essential that service users and other stakeholders are involved in the process. When preparing learners for clinical practice and to be registered health care practitioners the inclusion of service users is essential for the success of the programme. Experiences of receiving care must be contributed to improve the quality and standard of teaching and learning. Evaluation of care and of education is essential to identify where improvements need to be made.

Throughout curriculum and module development service users will be invited to contribute their experiences. Module leaders develop their content in relation to the curriculum design yet their methods and teaching techniques will vary. Including service users' experiences as learning material is hugely beneficial to the student and the module and it can have far-reaching positive effects on future experience. According to Atkinson and Williams (2011) it is essential that the process of curriculum development is discussed with service users so that the language used is clarified and their role in the process is defined. Service users are usually placed with academic and practice staff throughout the process to aid their understanding and promote their participation.

As part of student assessment many practice assessment documents include a section for service user feedback. Service users are often involved with assessments such as observed structured clinical examinations (OSCES). OSCES are used to assess a student's ability to simulate certain nursing skills. These are often very stressful assessments for students. However, with service user involvement, their stress can be reduced – the students feel that the client input lightens the situation (Atkinson and Williams, 2011). Students appreciate service user feedback to boost their confidence and confirm their competence.

Fitness to practise procedures

All education providers must have fitness to practise procedures to identify poor practice by student nurses in both academic and clinical practice. David and Lee-Woolf (2010) outline clearly the requirement for AEIs to have fitness to practise (FTP) procedures in place. The NMC control FTP for registered nurses and midwives, yet, as a student is still a learner and it is more appropriate for the university to establish FTP if concerns arise, a referral procedure should be available and all relevant staff in both the university and practice areas must be made aware of the processes required. Providing healthcare at learner level is deemed professional practice and therefore any misdemeanour within this practice must be investigated, with consequences afforded if proven. These include:

- Plagiarism
- Cheating and other dishonest behaviour
- Criminal conviction, caution, reprimand and penalty notice for disorder
- Unprofessional behaviour
- Substance misuse
- Health and mental health problems.

When discussing fitness to practise it is important to add that students need to learn about the potential consequences of not following the NMC Code (2018e). Education providers have a responsibility to educate students on the consequences of not adhering to the NMC Code and to the law. For qualified registered nurses, midwives and nursing associates the NMC (2018h) lists serious cases as:

- Cases involving dishonesty
- Cases involving sexual misconduct
- Cases involving criminal convictions or cautions.

--- **SCENARIO** ---

Fitness to practise

Nico is a Year 2 trainee nursing associate. He is on an eight-week place-ment on a respiratory ward. Nico has not been assigned many shifts with his supervisor and he is concerned that he will not be assessed appropri-ately due to this. Following discussion with his supervisor they decide that it would be okay for Nico to follow his supervisor on their shifts and not follow the ward allocation. There now is no ward record or evidence that Nico has been on placement. This arrangement is not approved by the ward manager and when Nico is not on shift the manager documents this and informs the university that Nico has been absent. When questioned by his personal tutor Nico insists that he was on placement with his supervisor and had the signatures to prove this in his practice assessment document. In his practice assessment document there were other dates that Nico insisted he was on placement when the ward manager did not see him. Following submission of these signatures on request by the programme leader and further discussion with the ward manager it is alleged that Nico has forged a number of signatures in his practice assessment document.

This is a fitness to practise issue and needs to be investigated by the appropriate university panel. It is a serious allegation and will have con-sequences for the trainee.

Every case will be assessed on its own merits. There may be a number of circumstances that need to be explored prior to a decision being made on any penalty for the trainee.

Can you identify a way that Nico and his supervisor could have made arrangements to work together legitimately? What do you think could be the outcome of this scenario? Consider the nursing and midwifery sanc-tions for their registered nurses, midwives and nursing associates. The NMC Code (2018e) outlines the responsibilities of the registered practi-tioner. When you consider the potential consequences for Nico please note that the trainee nursing associate is not yet a registered practitioner.

Being a professional indicates a level of responsibility within society. One way that a registered healthcare professional can demonstrate this is through their record keeping and documentation. Although examples of inadequate documentation and record keeping may not be directly considered a serious case when the NMC are considering sanctions in a hearing, it is highly likely that poor performance in relation to documentation could be viewed as dishonest behaviour. Dishonesty is most serious when a breach in the professional duty of candour is not approached openly and honestly when things go wrong in someone's care. Further information on documentation can be found later in this chapter.

Supporting students in various placement areas

The support of students in placement areas has a joint responsibility. Students will be provided with a supervisor, an assessor and an academic assessor in the placement area. However, the role of the education provider/university should also be present. In recent years placement areas have link tutors/link lecturers where the placement staff are visited on a regular basis for support with their students in practice. The student and the placement staff are the target of the linking and the visits, yet many link lecturers may also contribute with the development of the setting as a more effective learning environment (Gopee, 2018). Primarily the role is to link academic and clinical practice, with supervisors and assessors having access to the link in person or through other contact routes. While linking with an area the learners also have the opportunity to contact or to meet the link to raise any concerns relating to their learning but also to their general experience in the placement. For information related to the academic assessor please see Chapter 2.

ACTIVITY 5.3

Challenging behaviour

Read the following scenario then think through the questions below.

Samson is a student in your practice area and although he started his placement well, identified his learning objectives and the skills he expects to achieve during his placement, he has started to demonstrate some unacceptable behaviours in relation to communication with staff and with patients. It has been reported to you as Samson's practice assessor that staff have felt intimidated by him raising his voice, waving his arms and

(Continued)

walking away from discussions related to his behaviour. You have his midway assessment planned for the end of the week.

Questions

How do you plan to approach this change in behaviour?

Identify what support you require for this meeting?

Who could you include in your meeting for support?

What are you expecting from the individuals involved?

What does this mean for the future of Samson's placement?

Escalating concerns

As a supervisor and assessor to a student/learner in your care you need to be aware of how to raise any concerns that you or your student have with relation to protecting the public. All health providers will have a policy related to whistle blowing (please see Chapter 6).

There is guidance on raising concerns from the NMC (2017b) for nurses and midwives which identifies your role as the registered practitioner to guide your student on the steps to take and how to support them through the process with their education provider. All students must be supported by their education provider with regards to writing statements and providing evidence. It is important to remember that they are students, not employees and also not yet registered practitioners. Contact your link lecturer for any further advice related to policy and procedure.

ACTIVITY 5.4

Escalating concerns

Read the following scenario then think through the questions below.

Student nurse Tandy has been assigned to spend a number of shifts with registered nurse Michael in the operating department. Michael is very popular with staff and students. He is very helpful, good at teaching and sharing information. During break times Michael is very friendly and often shares his food with his colleagues and helps to create a fun, jovial atmosphere in the tea room.

Tandy has approached you as her supervisor to inform you that she has felt uncomfortable at times in Michael's presence. She reports to you that he comments on female patients' body types and on sexual acts he would like to participate in with these patients when they are under general anaesthesia. Although she does not want to believe that Michael has ever done anything with a patient, she is worried about patient safety. This has happened on more than one occasion and she feels that she needs to say something about it. When she has told Michael it is not appropriate to talk about patients in this manner he says he is only joking.

Questions

- What steps would you take to address this concern?
- What support can you offer Tandy? Who needs to be involved?
- What are the potential effects when this is escalated for you as the supervisor, for Tandy and for Michael?

Revalidation

Since April 2016 all registered nurses and midwives need to complete the process of revalidation every three years in order to remain active on the NMC register.

Revalidation was introduced to help you to demonstrate safe and effective practice. This new process replaces the Prep requirements and it is essential to renew your registration.

There are a number of requirements that need to be achieved and there are a number of resources available online through the NMC to assist you in achieving these (http://revalidation.nmc.org.uk/welcome-to-revalidation/index.html).

The requirements:

- 450 practice hours or 900 if renewing both as a nurse and a midwife
- 35 hours of CPD including 20 hours of participatory learning
- Five pieces of practice-related feedback
- Five written reflective accounts
- Reflective discussion

- Health and character declaration
- Professional indemnity arrangement
- Confirmation
- The payment of the registration fee (annually).

Although revalidation may appear to be a difficult task it is really quite straightforward and with the resources available it is highly achievable. Like many professional requirements it is advised that you gather the evidence and the information available to you throughout the three years prior to your revalidation. Doing this will inevitably make the task less onerous.

It is up to you as the registered professional to decide who your confirmer should be, although the NMC recommends that this is your line manager. Your confirmer will check whether or not the registered practitioner (nurse, midwife, nurse associate) has met the requirements of revalidation, complete your checks, and complete the NMC Confirmation Form for you to forward to the NMC as part of your revalidation process.

Documentation

The importance of documentation must never be underestimated. Correspondence needs to follow all of the correct principles in order to ensure consistency and accuracy in developing student nurses' performance. The Royal College of Nursing (2016) indicates the need to be honest, accurate and non-offensive and never breach patient confidentiality. Further recommendations are:

- Have legible handwriting or key in competently via electronic systems
- Always sign your entries
- Ensure entries are contemporaneous and dated and timed
- Record events clearly and accurately – remember that patients/clients/students may see this document at some point
- Keep factual – never speculate
- Avoid abbreviations or always explain them
- Record the patient's/client's/student's contribution to their care or, for a student, their observation/assessment
- Never alter another contributor's record
- When amending your documentation, draw a line through it and sign and date any changes
- Never write anything insulting or derogatory about any individual in your documentation.

Record keeping and documentation is a legal requirement for all registered personnel. We have all heard and used the line, 'if it's not written down, it didn't happen'. This statement is as important in relation to pre-registration students' progress as it is to patient care. The NMC Code (2018e) outlines the requirements for keeping clear and accurate records relevant to your practice for all nurses, midwives and nurse associates.

Supervisors and assessors need to document and record all interactions, learning opportunities, assessed skills, and formative and summative assessments in the student practice learning/assessment documents. Currently the majority of these documents are hard paper copies. In the future these will be electronic documents. This will enable ease of transfer of student learning records. All of the principles of documentation apply to recording your role with students. Remember we are protecting the public. Always be honest in your feedback and provide constructive criticism to your student. This will not only help the student improve but it will also inform the university and future supervisors and assessors of your student's progress. It is the responsibility of the practice assessor to ensure that all records and comments in the student's documentation are up to date and that any issues related to the performance of a student have been recorded and communicated with the next assessor and any other relevant people (NMC, 2018i).

Communication relating to student nurses is not only completed through their practice assessment/learning document. There are many ways with which we communicate with others relating to a student. This could be via email which follows all of the same principles of record keeping and documentation as outlined above. During telephone conversations with others always maintain your professionalism when discussing a student's performance.

ACTIVITY 5.5

Documentation

Read the example of an email below which references the following people then answer the questions below.

(Continued)

Zara Djani is the link tutor to Marmalade Ward.

Sarah Smith is a Year 3 student nurse on her penultimate placement on Marmalade Ward.

Patrice Brown is the student supervisor on Marmalade Ward.

Luigi Santana is the student assessor on Marmalade Ward.

Brenda Callaghan is the academic assessor for student nurse Sarah Smith.

From: Luigi Santana

Sent: 7 May 2020 10:09

To: Zara Djani

Subject: Sarah

Zara,

Need to let you know. Sarah has been late again today, she didn't ring to tell us she would be late. She keeps blaming her lateness on her own inability to sort out her childcare problems. When she is here, she is always untidy and looks dishevelled. I tried talking to her but she always turns on the water works and starts to cry. Me and Pat don't want to pass her on this placement. Patients like her but Sister has told me to let you know the problems. When are you coming to see us on the ward? Oh and can you tell Brenda as I can't find her contact details.

Ta, Lu

Questions

What do you think of the communication in this email/document?

What are the important parts of this email?

How would you consider rewriting this email?

How would you expect the link tutor to reply to this email correspondence?

CHAPTER SUMMARY

In this chapter we have:

- Explored the various education staff you could work with
- Considered what meetings you or others may be able to attend with the AEI
- Explored the role of education quality reviews/audits
- Considered why participation of service users in nursing education and assessment is important
- Discussed fitness to practise procedures at university level
- Considered how to escalate concerns of practice
- Provided information relating to nursing revalidation
- Discussed the importance of documentation.

6

STUDENT EMPOWERMENT

STANDARD 3

Student empowerment

S3.1 Students are provided with a variety of learning opportunities and appropriate resources which enable them to achieve their learning outcomes, NMC proficiencies and be capable of demonstrating the professional behaviours in *The Code*.

S3.2 Students are empowered and supported to become resilient, caring, reflective and lifelong learners who are capable of working in inter-professional and multi-agency teams.

AIMS OF THIS CHAPTER

- To understand how students learn
- To understand the different types of learner
- To understand the theories behind learning
- To understand what competency means, and how this affects practice
- To understand how to empower nurses and why this is important
- To understand the role of whistleblowing in healthcare and the procedures for this.

Introduction

It is important to appreciate that we all learn differently and have individual preferences that can aid and improve our learning. If our students have a particular learning style preference, then we can utilise this within the practice placement. You can find out what type of learner your student is by talking to them at your initial interview and asking some open questions.

- Ask your student what they have enjoyed in their practice placements so far? Why do they think this is?
- What has your student not enjoyed in their practice placements? Why do they think this is?
- How are they coping with the theory in their universities? Do they have any assignments or assessments outstanding?
- What do they want to achieve in this practice placement?

Students may have unrealistic expectations of their practice placement and this can be the time to discuss realistically what they will achieve during the time available. However, it is important as well to look for opportunities to stretch and challenge enthusiastic students. For example, you could encourage them to present a medical condition or they may like to research new medications and relate the pharmacology to the medical condition. Students who are cautious can be encouraged to take a more active role in the practice placement. Students who are struggling may have outstanding assignments or assessments or could be anxious about their progress and staying on top of their work. It is important to spend some time initially getting to know the students in this way so that you can support them in the most effective and appropriate way.

What type of learner are you?

Honey and Mumford identified four distinct types of learning: styles the activist, the pragmatist, the theorist, the reflector (Honey and Mumford, 1982. These are outlined in Figure 6.1.

ACTIVITY 6.1

Reflection on learning styles

Have you worked out what type of learner you are? How might you use this new knowledge to relate to your students?

Activists	Pragmatists
Activists are open minded, enthusiastic learners, they tend to act first and consider the consequences afterwards. They tackle problems by brainstorming. Activists thrive on challenges and activity but are bored by long-term consolidation.	Pragmatists are keen on innovative ideas, theories and techniques. They like to get on with things and act quickly, with a tendency to impatience. They tend to be practical down to earth people who view problems as a challenge.
Theorists	**Reflectors**
Theorists integrate observations into theories. They have a tendency towards perfection. They like to synthesise and analyse, and are keen to ask questions and challenge assumptions.	Reflectors like to observe from different perspectives. They like to gather information and think thoroughly before concluding. They are thoughtful and cautious and prefer to take a back seat.

Figure 6.1 Honey and Mumford's four learning styles

Learning theories

Understanding the theory behind learning is useful as it helps us to understand how to support our students and design learning experiences that aid this. We will now very briefly outline some of the key theories.

Andragogy

Knowles' theory of andragogy is aimed at adult learners whom he defined as having different properties than children. Adult learners are self-directed and bring experience to their learning environment. He outlined four principles of andragogy (esthermsmth, 2017).

- Adults are self-directed learners and should be involved in their learning and its content and design.
- Adults have past experience, and this should be utilised in their learning.
- Adults want practical learning, and content should be focused on work life.
- Learning should revolve round problem solving rather than memorising.

How can I use this theory with my student?

Adult learners have experience so find out what their experiences are and what they are bring to the practice placement. They may have very specific motivations for wanting to start a career as a healthcare professional or relevant experience providing care. Establishing prior experience can help you provide more effective learning opportunities for the student.

Key points

• Treat the student as an adult with respect for their life experiences, and do not treat them as children.

Humanist

At the heart of learning is the individual; their hopes, expectations and experiences. Abraham Maslow and Carl Rogers were leading proponents of humanism, which is a psychological approach that recognises the individual and their personal needs. When applied to education it is often termed as the student or learner centred approach.

Maslow's theory of self-actualisation suggests a pyramid of how we can achieve our full potential once basic needs are met (see Figure 6.2). These basic needs include physiological needs such as warmth and hunger. The second level includes safety needs such as shelter and security. Belonging needs come third and include the social needs to be part of a

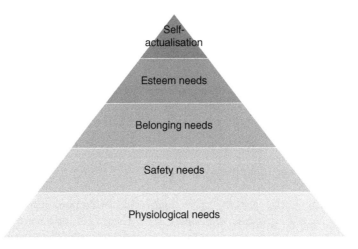

Figure 6.2 Maslow's hierarchy of needs (Maslow, 1943)

Source: Reproduced with permission of the American Psychological Association.

group. The next level is esteem needs, concerned with self-esteem, whilst at the top of the pyramid is self-fulfilment or self-actualisation.

Maslow and Rogers put the learner at the centre and encourage learners to take responsibility for their own learning.

How can I use this theory with my student?

Maslow's hierarchy of needs is useful as we sometimes forget students' physiological needs of hunger or tiredness which can result in their being less likely to retain information. If students feel unsafe, either with patients or within the environment, they may find it difficult to concentrate. Ensuring that students feel like they are a valued member of the healthcare team is important in order to ensure that they feel they are welcome and belong. Giving feedback, positive and constructive, can help to grow self-esteem, ultimately resulting in their professional self-actualisation. As educators we should consider whether the students who are excelling have been sufficiently challenged to reach their full potential; with weaker students we should consider whether we have helped to develop them sufficiently and ask ourselves if there other ways we can help them to reach their potential.

Key points

- Students are responsible for their learning.
- The educator's role is to help them achieve this by meeting their physiological and psychological needs, giving constructive feedback.
- Educators needs to acknowledge learners' personal experience and support self-directed learning.

Experiential learning theory

Kolb's experiential learning cycle (Figure 6.3) illustrates how reflection can be used to process experience and theory in order to develop. Drawing on concrete experiences we can reflect on our observations and review relevant abstract concepts and theory before attempting to put this learning into practice with active experimentation. Experiential learning is a continual and ever-changing process, and relies on reflection to analyse, gather and question the experience.

Active
Experimentation
Concrete
experience
Reflective
observation
Reviewing your
understanding of
abstract concepts

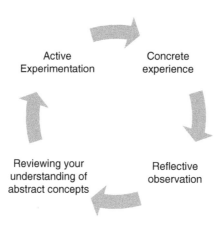

Figure 6.3 Kolb's experiential learning cycle

Source: © 2018 Experience Based Learning Systems, LLC. Reproduced with permission of Alice Kolb.

AN EXAMPLE OF KOLB'S EXPERIENTIAL LEARNING CYCLE IN ACTION

Figure 6.4 shows Kolb's learning cycle applied to a student learning how to perform an intramuscular injection.

Active experimentation
practising an intramuscular
injection e.g. with learning
resources
Concrete experience
performing the intramuscular
injection with a patient/client
Reflective observation
Reflecting what went well
and what did not go well
Reviewing your understanding
of abstract concepts Reviewing
why you do intramuscular
injections in the location you
do, and the risks of these

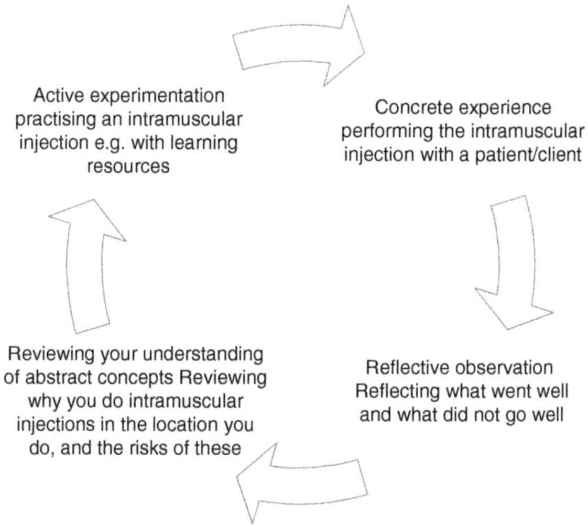

Figure 6.4 Kolb's learning in action

How can I use this theory with my student?

Students need to gain enough concrete experiences from their placements in order to learn experientially and this varies from person to person. Some individuals will need to observe and reflect more times than others to achieve the same level of learning. Useful experiences should generate problems, questions and thinking and this can be enhanced by activity, discussion and social interaction. Encouraging students to relate experiences to theoretical concepts and reflect through discussion and questioning can aid learning.

Reflection is a crucial component of experiential learning theory and can happen unconsciously and consciously. Reflection is enhanced by discussion and interacting with educators in the practice placement or in higher education institutes, so it is important to discuss, debate and question to encourage reflection. Learning how to reflect does not come naturally to all: students with the 'reflector' learning style are likely to find this skill easier to develop; activist and pragmatist learners on the other hand may need more support. You can support the student through regular meetings and appraisal of practice. Students must complete portfolios which require reflection and many struggle with these; you can support them by helping them to understand what is required, and encouraging them to reflect about clinical encounters. Reflection is a key component of professionalism and is required for revalidation of nursing registration. You can help your student learn to reflect by asking them to think about the experience and what went well.

- What would they do differently?
- How would they do this?
- What is the relevant theory connected with the experience?

You should then feedback on your observations of the encounter and what the student did well and could improve on. Encouraging the student to write this experience up will also aid reflection.

Key points

- Reflection is supported by active and challenging learning.
- Designing learning experiences that will aid learning is important.
- Reflection is the key to learning; supporting students to achieve this is vital for the development of professionalism.

Behaviourist

Behaviourism theorists include Skinner, Bandura, Watson, Pavlov and Thorndike and they assume that the learner is passive and a blank slate, with behaviour shaped through positive or negative reinforcement from their environment. Therefore, learning is determined by the environment and not by the individual learner. Critics of the model argue that it represents learning without understanding; however it remains a useful tool, particularly when teaching practical skills. An example of positive reinforcement is when parents reward good behaviour with treats or praise, and negative reinforcement would be where parents ignore children when they behave badly.

How can I use this theory with my student?

Behaviourist principles can be an effective way of teaching practical skills that require repetition and feedback. For example, handwashing has a clear objective and can be taught quickly then repeated with positive reinforcers to achieve good hand washing techniques.

Key points

- Educators should give clear objectives for the skill needed to be learnt.
- Reinforce the skill with positive and constructive feedback.

Social learning theory

Bandura's social learning theory argues that people learn from observing and imitating others. They can gain insight into how to act in different situations. The educator acts as a 'role model' and helps the student to rehearse how situations should be resolved. Positive role models are important to illustrate professionalism; however less experienced students may not possess enough knowledge at this stage of their training to be able to differentiate between poor and good role models. Role modelling is discussed in greater depth further in the chapter.

Key points

- Educators need to be aware of the effects of role modelling, even when they do not have an allocated student, as their behaviour and practice are observable.

Competency

Competency is the ability to work successfully and efficiently at an expected and defined level. Practice assessors and practice supervisors need to understand the level of competency expected for each level of nursing or other professional qualification. One of the integral parts of competency is the student recognising what they don't know and seeking help and support. Students who fail often don't have the ability to recognise where they are lacking knowledge and training; in other words, 'they don't know what they don't know' and this makes them unsafe.

It is important as a practice assessor that you are assessing the student at the expected level of attainment for their training and are not penalising as a result, perhaps, of expecting too much for their level of training. It is important that you know as a practice assessor what the students are expected to attain, and this is important even if they are pre-registered nurses or post-registered nurses. If you are unsure of the level of attainment expected of a student you are allocated, you should contact the academic supervisor or the module leader for the post-registered nursing course so that they can meet with you and discuss expectations. It is good practice for module leaders with post-registered courses with clinical placements to meet with practice assessors so that they understand the assessment requirements needed to be deemed competent.

Passing a student who is not competent may mean that an incompetent nurse is passed and allowed on the nursing register. For the practice assessor this may mean that the Nursing and Midwifery Council (NMC) may contact you if the nurse you have passed is found to be unsafe and you may be asked about your assessment of the nurse. The NMC will contact the academic supervisor as well as the practice assessor, asking about their assessment of the student. It is important to all registered nurses that they do not pass a nurse who is unsafe as this may affect their own nursing registration.

Do you know who your academic supervisor is? Have you met? Do you know the assessment requirements?

Role modelling

Role modelling is an important teaching tool for passing on knowledge, skills and values of professionalism. Role modelling is part of Bandura's social learning theory and is a tool used in nursing in practice placements. Students may experience positive and negative role models. Cruess et al. (2008) argue that health professionals need to analyse their performance as role models and be aware of the impact, both positive and negative, that role modelling can have. They believe that this can be achieved through protected time to facilitate dialogue, reflection and discussion with students, and by making a conscious effort to articulate the modelling which is implicit to them (Cruess et al., 2008).

ACTIVITY 6.2

Reflection on role models

What positive role models have influenced your career?

What negative role models have you come across? Why do you think these people were like this? How did it affect you?

Good role models encourage students to develop. They have high standards of nursing care, yet are caring and compassionate (see Figure 6.5). They show professionalism through the way they work, being punctual and maintaining confidentiality, yet working and communicating effectively within the clinical team. They are nurses who are moving the profession forward, developing their area of expertise and influencing the future. Poor role models may have poor clinical practice and may block development of others. They may lack knowledge or refuse to take on supervision of students, seeing them as a hindrance.

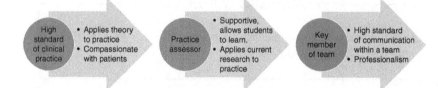

Figure 6.5   The qualities of a positive role model

NHS staff are expected to behave respectfully to patients, but sometime patients can be abusive, demonstrating behaviour that is unacceptable. Learning to cope with patients who are rude takes skill and experience that students may not yet possess and, therefore, how you act as a role model is very important. Burnell cautions nurses to be aware that patient rudeness 'is often a result of emotions or other factors which may not be obvious' (Burnell, 2015: 16) and this may negatively affect the care they receive. Burnell suggests that we use the Delude coping model to deal with patients who are rude (Burnell, 2015: 17).

————   THE DELUDE COPING MODEL   ————

D – Don't take it personally

E – Engage with the patient

L – Listen to the patient

U – Understand the problem and solution

D – Deal with it

E – Escalate the concern

Patients who are rude may feel that their concerns are not being heard, or may be scared. This simple model can help us to stop making premature judgements, reacting defensively or writing the patient off as a rude or 'difficult' person.

Whistleblowing

The NHS has produced guidelines on how to raise concerns about poor practice. Some concerns you might raise are:

- Unsafe patient care
- Unsafe working conditions
- Inadequate induction or training for staff
- Lack of, or poor, response to a reported patient safety incident
- Suspicions of fraud
- A bullying culture (across a team or organisation rather than individual instances of bullying).

(NHS Improvement, 2016: 4)

You may raise concerns confidentially and should not be victimised or harassed for raising a concern. Ideally you should raise concerns with your manager or tutor and report any adverse incident but, if this is not possible, you can speak directly to the Freedom To Speak Up Guardian (or equivalent designated person) or the hospital trust risk management team. Students can also feedback on practice assessors; an example can be seen in the next scenario.

──────────────── SCENARIO ────────────────

Raising concerns

Jess is a post-registered nurse undertaking a post-registered nursing course with a clinical placement. Her practice assessor Mary works with her on a one-to-one basis, teaching her in a clinic. Jess has noticed that Mary has given a patient a medication with patient group directives that may affect an existing liver disorder. Whilst it is not a contra-indication Jess realises that Mary should have sought a doctor's advice. Jess has also noticed that Mary has provided a medication to another patient without properly assessing the patient in the way the module leader has advised should be done.

Jess rings and speaks to her module leader Sue and discusses her experiences. She really likes Mary and does not want to get Mary into trouble.

Sue says that she will need to report the incidents to Mary's manager. She points out that patients are at risk and that she has a responsibility as a registered nurse to report the incident. Sue also asks Jess to write up the incident, which she does as well. She reminds Jess that she is a registered nurse and has a duty to report the incidents, but will support Jess throughout the process and find her another placement.

Sue reports the incident to Mary's manager, and finds that the manager has had concerns about Mary. The incidents are written up by Sue and Jess, and the manager meets with Mary to discuss the incidents.

It is important to remember that poor practice may have gone unnoticed because many health professionals work on their own with patients, for example, in community settings or clinics. This may mean that there is less direct observation of nurses' clinical practice and, as a result, a student may be the first to notice or question practice. Therefore we should always listen to students' concerns.

ACTIVITY 6.3

Peer review of team members

A good way to check clinical practice is to perform peer reviews of members of the nursing team. This can be an opportunity to give feedback on good practice as well as highlight poor practice. Feedback can be used for nurses' NMC revalidation.

Empowerment

Empowering students is vital for the development of intelligent, compassionate nurses. Empowering nurses to develop and reflect on their practice will help support this, but also encourage them to develop their career through writing articles and being involved in specialist organisations such as the RCN forum groups. Remember, these students represent the future workforce.

ACTIVITY 6.4

Reflection on empowerment

How can we empower nurses? What can you do to achieve this in your area?

Another way to empower nurses is to ensure that they are resilient. Lanz and Bruk-Lee (2017) found that highly resilient nurses bounced back after experiencing conflict in the workplace. They argued that we should explore resilience to reduce the negative effects of social stressors

(Lanz and Bruk-Lee, 2017). Recognising the importance of anxiety in nursing can help to improve resilience; the denial and depersonalisation of the significance of the individual patient to the nurse increases stress (Allan, 2016). We should recognise that some incidents are upsetting and give nurses time to debrief and value our professional role.

The next box offers some opportunities to empower nurses but you may have thought of others as the potential list is endless. The most important skill is to listen to the individual. What interests them? What do they want to do? If you can utilise their interest and passion then they are more likely to succeed as an educator.

POTENTIAL AREAS TO PROMOTE TO EMPOWER NURSES

Listen and find out what interests the individual and develop a plan to utilise this enthusiasm:

- Training that is relevant to expertise
- Theoretical courses (modules can often be put towards degree and master's programmes)
- Publication of module submissions, or commentaries, or discussion on new innovations in clinical practice
- Poster submission for conferences
- Representation on expert bodies and RCN forums
- Clinical supervision
- Coaching.

The last two points from the list are worth dwelling on. Clinical supervision is an excellent method to develop reflective techniques and encourage us to think about our clinical practice. Student nurses are taught this throughout their training. Clinical supervision helps to maintain safeguarding standards. It aids lifelong learning through clinical practice and the development of the practitioner's accountability. It is a method of support and influences personal and professional change (Driscoll, 2007). Coaching can be a long-term source of professional development for an individual. Coaching offers individualised support and the professional is seen as the expert, with the coach helping them to reach their full potential. It supports the individual to perform to their best, with the coach there to provide effective stimulation, ask good questions and provide guidance to help them identify the best solutions to problems.

In the current NHS climate, the support of clinical supervision and coaching is often neglected and the continuing development of future professionals is not regarded as a priority. This is a long-term approach which we neglect at our peril.

CHAPTER SUMMARY

In this chapter we have:

- Considered how students learn differently: understanding their learning style preferences will help support the way students learn
- Discussed how it is important not to pass a nurse who is not safe to practise
- Explored the concept of role models and how they are important influencers of students; we noted that there can be both positive and negative role models
- Looked at when to whistleblow and where your responsibility lies
- Considered how to empower nurses and looked at how coaching can help develop resilience.

APPENDIX 1

STANDARDS FRAMEWORK FOR NURSING AND MIDWIFERY EDUCATION

This appendix comes from part 1 of *Realising Professionalism: Standards for Education and Training* published 17 May 2018. It is an abridged version of *Part 1: Standards Framework for Education and Training*. The full standards are available at www.nmc.org.uk/standards-for-education-and-training.

1 Learning culture

Standards

1.1   The learning culture prioritises the safety of people, including carers, students and educators, and enables the values of *The Code* to be upheld.
1.2   Education and training is valued in all learning environments.

Requirements

Approved education institutions, together with practice learning partners, must:

1.1   demonstrate that the safety of people is a primary consideration in all learning environments

1.2   prioritise the wellbeing of people promoting critical self-reflection and safe practice in accordance with the *The Code*

1.3   ensure people have the opportunity to give and if required, withdraw, their informed consent to students being involved in their care

1.4   ensure educators and others involved in supervision, learning and assessment understand their role in preserving public safety

1.5   ensure students and educators understand how to raise concerns or complaints and are encouraged and supported to do so in line with local and national policies without fear of adverse consequences

1.6   ensure any concerns or complaints are investigated and dealt with effectively

1.7   ensure concerns or complaints affecting the wellbeing of people are addressed immediately and effectively

1.8   ensure mistakes and incidents are fully investigated and learning reflections and actions are recorded and disseminated

1.9   ensure students are supported and supervised in being open and honest with people in accordance with the professional duty of candour[1]

1.10 ensure the learning culture is fair, impartial, transparent, fosters good relations between individuals and diverse groups, and is compliant with equalities and human rights legislation[2]

1.11 promote programme improvement and advance equality of opportunity through effective use of information and data

1.12 ensure programmes are designed, developed, delivered, evaluated and co-produced with service users and other stakeholders

1.13 work with service providers to demonstrate and promote interprofessional learning and working, and

1.14 support opportunities for research collaboration and evidence-based improvement in education and service provision.

---

[1] www.nmc.org.uk/standards/guidance/the-professional-duty-of-candour

[2] www.equalityhumanrights.com/en/equality-act/equality-act-2010, in Northern Ireland www.equalityni.org

2 Educational governance and quality

Standards

2.1   There are effective governance systems that ensure compliance with all legal,[3] regulatory, professional and educational requirements, differentiating where appropriate between the devolved legislatures of the United Kingdom, with clear lines of responsibility and accountability for meeting those requirements and responding when standards are not met, in all learning environments.

2.2   All learning environments optimise safety and quality, taking account of the diverse needs of, and working in partnership with, service users, students and all other stakeholders.

Requirements

Approved education institutions, together with practice learning partners, must:

2.1   comply with all relevant legal, regulatory, professional and educational requirements

2.2   ensure programmes are designed to meet proficiencies and outcomes relevant to the programme

2.3   comply with NMC Programme standards specific to the programme being delivered

2.4   comply with NMC Standards for student supervision and assessment

2.5   adopt a partnership approach with shared responsibility for theory and practice supervision, learning and assessment, including clear lines of communication and accountability for the development, delivery, quality assurance and evaluation of their programmes

2.6   ensure that recruitment and selection of students is open, fair and transparent and includes measures to understand and address underrepresentation

2.7   ensure that service users and representatives from relevant stakeholder groups are engaged in partnership in student recruitment and selection

---

[3]Includes, but not limited to, relevant European Union legislation and legislation passed by devolved administrations of the United Kingdom.

2.8   demonstrate a robust process for recognition of prior learning (RPL) and how it has been mapped to the programme learning outcomes and proficiencies

2.9   provide students with the information and support they require in all learning environments to enable them to understand and comply with relevant local and national governance processes and policies

2.10 have robust, effective, fair, impartial and lawful fitness to practise procedures to swiftly address concerns about the conduct of students that might compromise public safety and protection

2.11 confirm that students meet the required proficiencies and programme outcomes in full, demonstrating their fitness for practice and eligibility for academic and professional award

2.12 provide all information and evidence required by regulators

2.13 regularly review all learning environments and provide assurance that they are safe and effective

2.14 have the capacity, facilities and resources in place to deliver safe and effective learning opportunities and practical experiences for students as required by their programme learning outcomes

2.15 be compliant with the NMC Standards for education and training[4] for all periods of learning undertaken outside the UK

2.16 improve quality, manage risk and disseminate effective practice through the proactive seeking and appropriate sharing of information and data

2.17 proactively identify and act on any areas for improvement, regularly measuring programme performance and outcomes against the NMC standards and requirements, and other recognised quality frameworks in education

2.18 appoint appropriately qualified and experienced people for programme delivery

2.19 identify programme leaders to confirm that all proficiencies have been met by each student by the end of their programme, and

2.20 ensure appropriately qualified and experienced external examiners consider and report on the quality of theory and practice learning.

---

[4]NMC Standards for education and training, standards established by NMC Council as necessary to achieve the standards of proficiency for admission to the register. Includes Parts 1, 2 and relevant standards in Part 3 and proficiencies.

3 Student empowerment

Standards

3.1   Students are provided with a variety of learning opportunities and appropriate resources which enable them to achieve proficiencies and programme outcomes and be capable of demonstrating the professional behaviours in *The Code*.

3.2   Students are empowered and supported to become resilient, caring, reflective and lifelong learners who are capable of working in inter-professional and inter-agency teams.

Requirements

Approved education institutions, together with practice learning partners, must ensure that all students:

3.1   have access to the resources they need to achieve the proficiencies and programme outcomes required for their professional role

3.2   are provided with timely and accurate information about curriculum, approaches to teaching, supervision, assessment, practice placements and other information relevant to their programme

3.3   have opportunities throughout their programme to work with and learn from a range of people in a variety of practice placements, preparing them to provide care to people with diverse needs

3.4   are enabled to learn and are assessed using a range of methods, including technology enhanced and simulation-based learning appropriate for their programme as necessary for safe and effective practice

3.5   are supervised and supported in practice learning in accordance with the NMC Standards for student supervision and assessment

3.6   are supervised according to their individual learning needs, proficiency and confidence

3.7   are allocated and can make use of supported learning time when in practice

3.8   are assigned and have access to a nominated practice assessor for a practice placement or a series of practice placements in addition to a nominated academic assessor for each part of the education programme, in accordance with the NMC Standards for student supervision and assessment

3.9   have the necessary support and information to manage any interruptions to the study of programmes for any reason

3.10   are provided with timely and accurate information regarding entry to NMC registration or annotation of their award

3.11   have their diverse needs respected and taken into account across all learning environments, with support and adjustments provided in accordance with equalities and human rights legislation and good practice

3.12   are protected from discrimination, harassment and other behaviour that undermines their performance or confidence

3.13   are provided with information and support which encourages them to take responsibility for their own mental and physical health and wellbeing

3.14   are provided with the learning and pastoral support necessary to empower them to prepare for independent, reflective professional practice

3.15   are well prepared for learning in theory and practice having received relevant inductions

3.16   have opportunities throughout their programme to collaborate and learn with and from other professionals, to learn with and from peers, and to develop supervision and leadership skills

3.17   receive constructive feedback throughout the programme from stakeholders with experience of the programme to promote and encourage reflective learning, and

3.18   have opportunities throughout their programme to give feedback on the quality of all aspects of their support and supervision in both theory and practice.

4 Educators and assessors

Standard

4.1   Theory and practice learning and assessment are facilitated effectively and objectively by appropriately qualified and experienced professionals with necessary expertise for their educational and assessor roles.

Requirements

Approved education institutions, together with practice learning partners, must ensure that all educators and assessors:

4.1   comply with all standards and requirements in the *NMC Standards for education and training*

4.2   act as professional role models at all times

4.3   receive relevant induction, ongoing support and access to education and training which includes training in equality and diversity

4.4   have supported time and resources to enable them to fulfil their roles in addition to their other professional responsibilities

4.5   respond effectively to the learning needs of individuals

4.6   are supportive and objective in their approach to student supervision and assessment

4.7   liaise and collaborate with colleagues and partner organisations in their approach to supervision and assessment

4.8   are expected to respond effectively to concerns and complaints about public protection and student performance in learning environments and are supported in doing so

4.9   receive and act upon constructive feedback from students and the people they engage with to enhance the effectiveness of their teaching, supervision and assessment

4.10   share effective practice and learn from others, and

4.11   appropriately share and use evidence to make decisions on student assessment and progression.

5 Curricula and assessment

Standard

5.1 Curricula and assessments are designed, developed, delivered and evaluated to ensure that students achieve the proficiencies and outcomes for their approved programme.

Requirements

Approved education institutions, together with practice learning partners, must ensure:

5.1 curricula fulfil NMC Programme standards, providing learning opportunities that equip students to meet the proficiencies and programme outcomes[5]

5.2 curricula remain relevant in respect of the contemporary health and social care agenda

5.3 curricula weigh theory and practice learning appropriately to the programme

5.4 curricula are developed and evaluated by suitably experienced and qualified educators and practitioners who are accountable for ensuring that the curriculum incorporates relevant programme outcomes

5.5 curricula are co-produced with stakeholders who have experience relevant to the programme

5.6 curricula provide appropriate structure and sequencing that integrates theory and practice at increasing levels of complexity

5.7 curricula are structured and sequenced to enable students to manage their theory and practice learning experience effectively

5.8 assessment is fair, reliable and valid to enable students to demonstrate they have achieved the proficiencies for their programme

5.9 adjustments are provided in accordance with relevant equalities and human rights legislation for assessments in theory and practice

5.10 students are assessed across practice settings and learning environments as required by their programme

---

[5]Applies equally to all programmes whether delivered as full time or less than full time.

5.11   assessment is mapped to the curriculum and occurs throughout the programme to determine student progression

5.12   practice assessment is facilitated and evidenced by observations and other appropriate methods

5.13   students' self-reflections contribute to, and are evidenced in, assessments

5.14   a range of people including service users contribute to student assessment

5.15   assessment of practice and theory is weighted appropriately to the programme, and

5.16   there is no compensation in assessments across theory and practice learning.

APPENDIX 2

STANDARDS FOR STUDENT SUPERVISION AND ASSESSMENT

This appendix comes from part 2 of *Realising Professionalism: Standards for Education and Training* published 17 May 2018. It is an abridged version of *Part 2: Standards for Student Supervision and Assessment*. The full standards are available at www.nmc.org.uk/standards-for-education-and-training.

Effective practice learning

All students are provided with safe, effective and inclusive learning experiences. Each learning environment has the governance and resources needed to deliver education and training.

Students actively participate in their own education, learning from a range of people across a variety of settings.

1. Organisation of practice learning

Approved education institutions, together with practice learning partners must ensure that:

1.1   practice learning complies with the NMC *Standards framework for nursing and midwifery education*

1.2   practice learning complies with specific programme standards
1.3   practice learning is designed to meet proficiencies and outcomes relevant to the programme
1.4   there are suitable systems, processes, resources and individuals in place to ensure safe and effective coordination of learning within practice learning environments
1.5   there is a nominated person for each practice setting to actively support students and address student concerns
1.6   students are made aware of the support and opportunities available to them within all learning environments
1.7   students are empowered to be proactive and to take responsibility for their learning
1.8   students have opportunities to learn from a range of relevant people in practice learning environments, including service users, registered and non-registered individuals, and other students as appropriate
1.9   learning experiences are inclusive and support the diverse needs of individual students
1.10   learning experiences are tailored to the student's stage of learning, proficiencies and programme outcomes, and
1.11   all nurses, midwives and nursing associates contribute to practice learning in accordance with *The Code*.

Supervision of students

Practice supervision enables students to learn and safely achieve proficiency and autonomy in their professional role. All NMC registered nurses, midwives and nursing associates are capable of supervising students, serving as role models for safe and effective practice. Students may be supervised by other registered health and social care professionals.

2. Expectations of practice supervision

Approved education institutions, together with practice learning partners, must ensure that:

2.1   all students on an NMC approved programme are supervised while learning in practice
2.2   there is support and oversight of practice supervision to ensure safe and effective learning

2.3   the level of supervision provided to students reflects their learning needs and stage of learning

2.4   practice supervision ensures safe and effective learning experiences that uphold public protection and the safety of people

2.5   there is sufficient coordination and continuity of support and supervision of students to ensure safe and effective learning experiences

2.6   practice supervision facilitates independent learning, and

2.7   all students on an NMC approved programme are supervised in practice by NMC registered nurses, midwives, nursing associates and other registered health and social care professionals.

3. Practice supervisors: role and responsibilities

Approved education institutions, together with practice learning partners, must ensure that practice supervisors:

3.1   serve as role models for safe and effective practice in line with their code of conduct

3.2   support learning in line with their scope of practice to enable the student to meet their proficiencies and programme outcomes

3.3   support and supervise students, providing feedback on their progress towards, and achievement of, proficiencies and skills

3.4   have current knowledge and experience of the area in which they are providing support, supervision and feedback, and

3.5   receive ongoing support to participate in the practice learning of students.

4. Practice supervisors: contribution to assessment and progression

Approved education institutions, together with practice learning partners, must ensure that practice supervisors:

4.1   contribute to the student's record of achievement by periodically recording relevant observations on the conduct, proficiency and achievement of the students they are supervising

4.2   contribute to student assessments to inform decisions for progression

4.3   have sufficient opportunities to engage with practice assessors and academic assessors to share relevant observations on the conduct, proficiency and achievement of the students they are supervising, and

4.4   are expected to appropriately raise and respond to student conduct and competence concerns and are supported in doing so.

5. Practice supervisors: preparation

Approved education institutions, together with practice learning partners, must ensure that practice supervisors:

5.1   receive ongoing support to prepare, reflect and develop for effective supervision and contribution to, student learning and assessment, and

5.2   have understanding of the proficiencies and programme outcomes they are supporting students to achieve.

Assessment of students and confirmation of proficiency

Student assessments are evidence based, robust and objective. Assessments and confirmation of proficiency are based on an understanding of student achievements across theory and practice. Assessments and confirmation of proficiency are timely, providing assurance of student achievements and competence.

6. Assessor roles

Approved education institutions, together with practice learning partners, must ensure that:

6.1   all students on an NMC approved programme are assigned to a different nominated academic assessor for each part of the education programme

6.2   all students on an NMC approved programme are assigned to a nominated practice assessor for a practice placement or a series of practice placements, in line with local and national policies

6.3   nursing students are assigned to practice and academic assessors who are registered nurses with appropriate equivalent experience for the student's field of practice

6.4   midwifery students are assigned to practice and academic assessors who are registered midwives

6.5   specialist community public health nurse (SCPHN) students are assigned to practice and academic assessors who are registered SCPHNs with appropriate equivalent experience for the student's field of practice

6.6   nursing associate students are assigned to practice and academic assessors who are either a registered nursing associate or a registered nurse

6.7   students studying for an NMC approved post-registration qualification are assigned to practice and academic assessors in accordance with relevant programme standards

6.8   practice and academic assessors receive ongoing support to fulfil their roles, and

6.9   practice and academic assessors are expected to appropriately raise and respond to concerns regarding student conduct, competence and achievement, and are supported in doing so.

7. Practice assessors: responsibilities

Approved education institutions, together with practice learning partners, must ensure that:

7.1   practice assessors conduct assessments to confirm student achievement of proficiencies and programme outcomes for practice learning

7.2   assessment decisions by practice assessors are informed by feedback sought and received from practice supervisors

7.3   practice assessors make and record objective, evidenced-based assessments on conduct, proficiency and achievement, drawing on student records, direct observations, student self-reflection, and other resources

7.4   practice assessors maintain current knowledge and expertise relevant for the proficiencies and programme outcomes they are assessing

7.5   a nominated practice assessor works in partnership with the nominated academic assessor to evaluate and recommend the student for progression for each part of the programme, in line with programme standards and local and national policies

7.6   there are sufficient opportunities for the practice assessor to periodically observe the student across environments in order to inform decisions for assessment and progression

7.7   there are sufficient opportunities for the practice assessor to gather and coordinate feedback from practice supervisors, any other practice assessors, and relevant people, in order to be assured about their decisions for assessment and progression

7.8   practice assessors have an understanding of the student's learning and achievement in theory

7.9   communication and collaboration between practice and academic assessors is scheduled for relevant points in programme structure and student progression

7.10   practice assessors are not simultaneously the practice supervisor and academic assessor for the same student, and

7.11   practice assessors for students on NMC approved prescribing programmes support learning in line with the NMC Standards for prescribing programmes.

8. Practice assessors: preparation

Approved education institutions, together with practice learning partners, must ensure that practice assessors:

8.1   undertake preparation or evidence prior learning and experience that enables them to demonstrate achievement of the following minimum outcomes:

  8.1.1 interpersonal communication skills, relevant to student learning and assessment

  8.1.2 conducting objective, evidence based assessments of students

  8.1.3 providing constructive feedback to facilitate professional development in others, and

  8.1.4 knowledge of the assessment process and their role within it

8.2   receive ongoing support and training to reflect and develop in their role

8.3   continue to proactively develop their professional practice and knowledge in order to fulfil their role, and

8.4   have an understanding of the proficiencies and programme outcomes that the student they assess is aiming to achieve.

9. Academic assessors: responsibilities

Approved education institutions, together with practice learning partners, must ensure that:

9.1   academic assessors collate and confirm student achievement of proficiencies and programme outcomes in the academic environment for each part of the programme

9.2   academic assessors make and record objective, evidence-based decisions on conduct, proficiency and achievement, and recommendations for progression, drawing on student records and other resources

9.3   academic assessors maintain current knowledge and expertise relevant for the proficiencies and programme outcomes they are assessing and confirming

9.4   the nominated academic assessor works in partnership with a nominated practice assessor to evaluate and recommend the student for progression for each part of the programme, in line with programme standards and local and national policies

9.5   academic assessors have an understanding of the student's learning and achievement in practice

9.6   communication and collaboration between academic and practice assessors is scheduled for relevant points in programme structure and student progression, and

9.7   academic assessors are not simultaneously the practice supervisor and practice assessor for the same student.

10. Academic assessors: preparation

Approved education institutions, together with practice learning partners, must ensure that academic assessors:

10.1   are working towards or hold relevant qualifications as required by their academic institution and local and national policies

10.2   demonstrate that they have achieved the following minimum outcomes:

10.2.1   interpersonal communication skills, relevant to student learning and assessment

10.2.2   conducting objective, evidence based assessments of students

10.2.3   providing constructive feedback to facilitate professional development in others, and

10.2.4   knowledge of the assessment process and their role within it

10.3   receive ongoing support and training to reflect and develop in their role

10.4   continue to proactively develop their professional practice and knowledge in order to fulfil their role, and

10.5   have an understanding of the proficiencies and programme outcomes that the student they confirm is aiming to achieve.

REFERENCES

Allan, H. (2016) 'Editorial: The anxiety of caring and the devalue of nursing', *Journal of Clinical Nursing*. https://doi:10.1111/jocn.13380

Atkinson, S. and Williams, P. (2011) 'The involvement of service users in nursing students' education', *Learning Disability Practice*, 14 (3): 18–21.

Burnell, R.I. (2015) 'The right to be rude: managing of conflict', *Nursing Times*, 112 (1/2): 16–19.

Calkin, S. (2011) 'Whistleblowing Mid Staffs nurse too scared to walk to car after shift', *Nursing Times*, 17 October.

Chan, D.S. (2004) 'Nursing students' perceptions of hospital learning environments: an Australian perspective', *International Journal of Nursing Education Scholarship*, 1 (1). **DOI:** https://doi.org/10.2202/1548-923X.1002

Cruess, S.R., Cruess, R.L. and Steinert, Y. (2008) 'Role modelling: making the most of a powerful teaching strategy', *BMJ* 336. doi: https://doi.org/10.1136/bmj.39503.757847.BE

David, T.J. and Lee-Woolf, E. (2010) 'Fitness to practise for student nurses: principles, standards and procedures', *Nursing Times*. www.nursingtimes.net/roles/district-and-community-nurses/fitness-to-practise-for-student-nurses-principles-standards-and-procedures/5020031.article [accessed 27 November 2018]

Department of Health (2014) *Introducing the Statutory Duty of Candour*. London: Department of Health.

Driscoll, J. (2007) *Practising Clinical Supervision*. London: Bailliere Tindall.

Duffy, K. (2003) *Failing Students: A Qualitative Study of Factors that Influence the Decisions Regarding Assessment of Students' Competence in Practice*. Glasgow: Glasgow Caledonian University.

Duffy, K (2013) 'Providing constructive feedback to students during mentoring', *Nursing Standard*, 27 (31): 50–6.

Elcock, K. and Sharples, K. (2011) *A Nurse's Survival Guide to Mentoring*. London: Elsevier.

Emanuel, V. (2013) 'Creating supportive environments for students', *Nursing Times*, 109 (37): 18–20.

esthermsmth (2017) 'Andragogy – adult learning theory (Knowles)', *Learning Theories*, 30 Sept. www.learning-theories.com/andragogy-adult-learning-theory-knowles.htm [accessed 11 April. 2018]

Francis, R. (2013) *The Francis Report*. London. Mills & Reeve.

General Medical Council (2013) *Good Medical Practice*. London: GMC.

Gibbs, G. (1988) *Learning by Doing: A Guide to Teaching and Learning Methods*. Oxford: Oxford Further Education Unit.

Gillen, S. (2013) 'Former Mid Staffs director denies 29 breaches of NMC code', *Nursing Standard*, 27 (48): 11.

Gopee, N. (2018) *Supervision and Mentoring in Healthcare*, 4th ed. London: Sage.

Honey, P. and Mumford, A. (1982) *Manual of Learning Styles*. London: P. Honey.

Hughes, S. and Quinn, F.M. (2013) *Quinn's Principles and Practice of Nurse Education*, 6th ed. Andover: Cengage.

Jones-Barry, S. (2018) 'Why nursing students leave: the truth about attrition', *Nursing Standard*, 33 (9): 14–16.

Kolb, A. (2014) *Experiential Learning: Experience as the Source of Learning and Development, 2nd ed.* New York: Pearson FT Press.

Lanz, J.L. and Bruk-Lee, V. (2017) 'Resilience as a moderator of the indirect effects of conflict and workload on job outcomes among nurses', *Journal of Advanced Nursing*, 73: 2973–86.

Maslow (1943) 'A Theory of Human Motivation' *Psychological Review*, 50: 370–396.

NHS Improvement (2016) *Freedom to Speak up: Raising Concerns (Whistle-blowing) Policy for the NHS*. NHS Improvement (April). Publication code: Policy 01/16 Publications Gateway Reference: 04877. England.

NHS Improvement (2018). *Freedom to Speak up: Guidance for NHS Trust and NHS Foundation Trust Boards*. NHS Improvement: England.

NMC (2006) *Standards to Support Learning Assessment in Practice*. London: NMC.

NMC (2008) *Standards to Support Learning and Assessment in Practice NMC Standards for Mentors, Practice Teachers and Teachers*. London: NMC.

NMC (2010a) *Standards for Pre-Registration Nursing Education*. London: NMC.

NMC (2010b) *Standards for Competence for Registered Nurses*. London: NMC.

NMC (2017a) 'New figures show an increase in numbers of nurses and midwives leaving the profession', *NMC*, 3 July.

NMC (2017b) *Raising Concerns: Guidance for Nurses and Midwives*. London: NMC.

NMC (2018a) *Realising Professionalism: Standards for Education and Training. Part 1: Standards Framework for Nursing and Midwifery Education*. London: NMC.

NMC (2018b) *Realising Professionalism: Standards for Education and Training. Part 2: Standards for Student Supervision and Assessment*. London: NMC.

NMC (2018c) *Realising Professionalism: Standards for Education and Training. Part 3: Standards for Pre-Registration Nursing Programmes*. London: NMC.

NMC (2018d) *Future Nurse: Standards of Proficiency for Registered Nurses*. London: NMC.

NMC (2018e) *The Code: Professional Standards of Practice and Behaviour for Nurses, Midwives and Nursing Associates*. London: NMC.

NMC (2018f) 'Striking off order.' www.nmc.org.uk/ftp-library/sanctions/the-sanctions/striking-off-order/ [accessed 27 December 2018].

NMC (2018g) *Quality Assurance Framework for Nurses, Midwives and Nursing Associate Education.* London: NMC.

NMC (2018h) 'Considering sanctions for serious cases SAN-2.' www.nmc.org.uk/ftp-library/sanctions/sanctions-serious-cases/ [accessed 24 January 2019].

NMC (2018i) 'Handing over to the next assessor', PA3-D. www.nmc.org.uk/supporting-information-on-standards-for-student-supervision-and-assessment/practice-assessment/what-do-practice-assessors-do/handing-over-to-the-next-assessor/ [accessed 24 January 2019].

Paley, J. (2014) 'Cognition and the compassion deficit: the social psychology of helping behaviour in nursing', *Nursing Philosophy*, 15 (4) 274–287.

Royal College of Nursing (2016) 'Principles of record keeping.' https://rcni.com/hosted-content/rcn/first-steps/principles-of-record-keeping [accessed 24 January 2019].

Royal College of Nursing (2017a) *RCN Guidance for Mentors of Nursing and Midwifery.* London: RCN.

Royal College of Nursing (2017b) *The UK Nursing Labour Market Review 2017.* London: RCN.

Somerville, C. (2015) *Unhealthy Attitudes: The Treatment of LGBT People within Health and Social Care Services.* London: Stonewall.

Walsh, D. (2014) *The Nurse Mentor's Handbook, Supporting Students in Clinical Practice*, 2nd ed. Maidenhead, Berks: OU Press.

INDEX

Page references to Figures contain the letter 'f', whereas references to Tables are followed by the letter 't'.